The Emotional First + Aid Kit

A Practical Guide to Life After

Bariatric Surgery

Second Edition

by Cynthia L. Alexander, PsyD

Matrix Medical Communications

The Emotional First + Aid Kit
A Practical Guide to Life After Bariatric Surgery
Second Edition

Matrix Medical Communications
1595 Paoli Pike, Suite 103
West Chester, PA 19380

President/Group Publisher: Robert L. Dougherty
Partner: Patrick Scullin
Vice President, Publisher: Joseph J. Morris
Vice President, Editorial Director: Elizabeth A. Klumpp
Executive Editor: Kimberly B. Chesky
Senior Managing Editor: Colleen M. Hutchinson
Assistant Editor: Angela M. Hayes

Printed in the United States.

ISBN 978-0-9768526-5-0

Note from the publisher: *This book provides basic information about a broad range of medical conditions. It is not intended to serve as a tool for diagnosing illness, in prescribing treatments, or as a substitute for the physician/patient relationship. All persons concerned about medical symptoms or the possibility of disease are encouraged to seek professional care from an appropriate healthcare provider.*

To Leslie

For her ability to magically transform
the impossible into reality

The Emotional First + Aid Kit
A Practical Guide to Life After Bariatric Surgery
Second Edition

- Family anger
- Abuse
- Others concerned with your weight

This book's purpose is to help all those wishing to change their lives through bariatric/gastric bypass surgery. As a psychologist, I have seen hundreds of people both before and after surgery and have witnessed firsthand their problems and trials, as well as their successes. In this book, we will discuss many of the difficulties a bariatric patient is likely to encounter and some realistic and practical strategies for dealing with them. Most people go into bariatric surgery full of motivation and hope, only to find day-to-day postoperative existence more stressful than they imagined. Here are the psychological tricks of the trade to help make your own journey a successful one.

Your Mind is Your Most Important Weapon

I f you are considering bariatric surgery, or have had the surgery, you are facing one of the biggest challenges you will encounter in your lifetime. Few other decisions will be so life-altering and transformational. The surgery is irreversible, except in the rarest and most dire of circumstances.

Bariatric surgery is often referred to by healthcare providers as a "tool" to help you achieve your weight loss goals. This is realistic in regards to weight loss, but many people believe it is much more than that. Try to think of it as an "assistant," rather than a tool as this more accurately describes its role. Many people tend to believe it is the magic pill for which they have been waiting. In reality, life after surgery is very much like living with a very strict diet and exercise plan, just like a traditional diet. All the struggles and temptations that you must master on traditional diet and exercise plans are still there for you to contend with in the years following surgery.

The surgery does not force a person to change. Initially, there will likely be ramifications if the diet is not followed, but eventually these will diminish. Long-term diet and exercise changes are the key to success after surgery, but the surgery will not make these changes happen.

The importance of having realistic expectations cannot be overstated. Those that truly understand what the surgery does and does not provide will have better results.

Many patients come to my office prior to surgery and say, "This surgery will help me because I won't be able to cheat." This is an unrealistic expectation. You can cheat just like on any other diet program. The reality is that most people lose weight for the first six months because it is usually difficult to eat. But just like with a traditional diet, you must watch what you eat and exercise regularly in order to be successful.

It is very important to remember that the surgery component is separate from the lifestyle change component. The lifestyle change involves both regular exercise for life and strict dietary changes. The bonus

THE SURGERY DOES NOT FORCE a person to change...Long-term diet and exercise changes are the key to success after surgery, but the surgery will not make these changes happen.

THE BONUS OF THE SURGERY is that you lose weight rapidly if you follow the diet given by the surgeon—the idea being that rapid weight loss will keep you motivated so you will stick with the diet and exercise as you see results.

of the surgery is that you lose weight rapidly if you follow the diet given by the surgeon—the idea being that rapid weight loss will keep you motivated so you will stick with the diet and exercise as you see results. It will also assist in maintaining the weight loss if you follow the guidelines for life. You will feel full with much less food, and for those with weight-related health problems, such as diabetes, sleep apnea, and high blood pressure, this can be a life-saving surgery.

In this book, I will attempt to provide information acquired over many years in the field of bariatric psychology. Whether you have already had the surgery, are planning to have it, or are still undecided, this information can benefit you in both your weight loss and weight maintenance goals.

This second edition contains new information. Every year we learn more about the long-term results of bariatric surgery. Much of the information is positive, including the exciting studies that show diabetes is resolved in more than 80 percent of cases for those choosing gastric bypass. Some of the information is negative, including new information on severe depression and transfer of addiction. It is my hope that by reading these chapters, well-educated patients will be able to make good decisions on their own behalf.

This book is intended as a reference and may be helpful in identifying and addressing certain problems facing bariatric surgery patients. Some people think of the book as a "pocket psychologist." Just like a medical manual, certain problems can be addressed by following simple instructions, but for more serious issues you would be directed to see a physician. Similarly, many solutions will be offered in this book, but for more serious issues that could lead to eating disorders, depression, or suicide, it may be necessary to see your own psychologist. This book will teach you to recognize when you may have a serious problem and when it is appropriate to get involved in regular therapy with a psychologist.

In this book, several main themes will be discussed in many different ways and can have great impact on your ability to be successful after surgery:

A. Stress, how it affects your ability to stick with dietary changes and exercise, and what to do about it

B. How we are our own worst enemy when it comes to lifestyle changes and how to gain control

C. Self-talk, what it is, how it works, and how you can use it to help you with eating and exercise

D. Successful habits used by successful patients.

As you lose weight, you will likely experience many psychological and physical changes. This is your chance at a new beginning, and what that beginning entails is entirely up to you. For some, it means a new wardrobe. For others, it means a new career, a new boyfriend or girlfriend, or a chance at a higher quality of life. Even more importantly, it can mean a chance to decrease disease and medication use. The important point is to do what is right for you and for the right reasons. Talk about your situation with friends, family, or a psychologist.

One of my star patients told me she feels as though the day she had her surgery, she was "reborn." She calls herself a "toddler" after having the surgery four years ago. Her rationale is that toddlers have learned much about themselves and their own motivations and still

> # THE MOST IMPORTANT DIFFERENCE
> between those who are successful and those who regain weight is the proper use of psychology.

have so much to learn. People who had surgery last month will be learning many new things about themselves every day, much like an infant. She often counsels others to be patient with themselves. After all, it takes many years to unlearn old habits and to get used to the new you. The surgeons agree. I hear them say to patients, "We operate on your stomach, not your head." Bariatric surgery is a wonderful tool, but the rest is up to you.

WHY DO I NEED PSYCHOLOGY AFTER SURGERY?

Many people wonder why psychology is even important. After all, most people will lose a significant amount of weight after surgery. The answer is that psychology helps us to do what we know we should when we have trouble doing it on our own. For example, we all know it is important to eat foods in moderation and to exercise, but do we do it? Of course not. Similarly, after surgery there will be lists of foods you should eat and those you should avoid. There will be suggestions on how often to exercise and lists of vitamins you should take as well. In the beginning, it is easier to follow the set guidelines, but people often struggle with them as time goes on. This is when good psychological tips and techniques can make the difference between success and failure.

The main weapon in your arsenal for weight loss success is your mind. With it, you will learn to change the thoughts that keep you from being successful, and use it to establish new habits for life. This time will be different. This time you will not lose the weight just to gain it back again. The most important difference between those who are successful and those who regain weight is the proper use of psychology. If you combine what you learn in this book with the advice of your program's dietitian, surgeon, and others, you will be successful. You will use your mind to change your behaviors and to look at your environment for obstacles to success. Up until now your mind may have worked against you, but starting today, you will be in charge. Starting today, you will begin to learn the techniques and gain the psychological tools that will take you through weight loss and on to weight maintenance for life.

The Decision to Have Bariatric Surgery

ariatric surgery itself will vary from program to program and from surgeon to surgeon. There are several different bypass surgeries, and they may be done open or laparoscopically. There are banding procedures as well. While the procedures, risks, and benefits to each one may vary, the lifestyle changes required for long-term success are similar. Each procedure will require long-term dietary changes and exercise for life. The first step is to decide if surgery is right for you.

PROS AND CONS

How do you make a decision that will affect you for the rest of your life? Few decisions you will ever make are as permanent as the decision to have bariatric surgery, much like the decision to have children. Most patients tell me that they agonized over the decision for months or even years before going ahead with it. It is important to look at this realistically in order to make an informed decision. That includes looking closely at all the risks and benefits, including the risk of death, and asking yourself if it is worth that kind of personal risk.

Bariatric surgery can be life saving, but it requires effort, commitment, and responsibility on the part of the patient for long-term success. How do you know if you are ready for the effort and responsibility?

A tried and true psychological method to help make an important decision is to list the pros and cons; therefore, it is a very good idea for patients to list the pros and cons of having the surgery and the pros and cons of not having the surgery. The only catch is that you must be honest and realistic with your answers.

✐ ACTIVITY—THE PROS AND CONS GRAPH

Step 1: On a piece of paper, draw a large box and divide it into four equal squares. Label each box as follows: Pros of having surgery (upper left box); cons of having surgery (upper right box); pros of not having surgery (lower left box); and cons of not having surgery (lower right box) (see next page).

Now concentrate on one box at a time and make a comprehensive list for each one. Be really honest with yourself, and list everything that comes to mind. It is important to list benefits of not having the surgery, such as less stress, being able to enjoy your favorite celebration rituals involving food, or not having to exercise. Examples of pros for having the surgery are increased mobility and increased self

Pros of having surgery	Cons of having surgery
Pros of not having surgery	Cons of not having surgery

Pros and Cons Graph

esteem. Take some time to think about this in detail, and write it all down.

Once you have completed this, one box will make more sense to you than the others. It may not be your first choice, but this box may represent the best choice for you.

If your best choice turns out to be to not have the surgery, this may simply mean you really crave weight loss, but are not ready to make the drastic changes that come with bariatric surgery. If this is the case, just wait a few months, and try the pros and cons graph again. Your success with the surgery depends on the dietary and exercise changes you must make, so you need to be sure you are

Case Study

Jim came to the hospital using a walker and was barely able to walk down the short hallway to my office. By the time he sat down, he was breathing heavily and was exhausted. He explained that since he had been diagnosed with diabetes and gained the last 50 pounds, his health had steadily deteriorated. It was evident that Jim was finding it difficult to function in his everyday life, and his future looked bleak.

Of course the risks were worrisome to Jim. He said, "It's only going to get worse if I don't do something about this weight." He was unable to exercise due to severe joint pain. He knew he would have to reduce his weight somehow without exercise, and start slowly when his weight decreased to the point when he could move without a walker.

Jim had the surgery, and five months later I saw him at a meeting. He had lost over 100 pounds and was not using a walker. He explained he had started walking and was up to two miles a day. He appeared to be happier, and his health had definitely improved.

Jim's decision to have the surgery was literally to save his life. He told me later the surgery had been a miracle that gave him a "second chance" and that he did not intend to waste that chance.

committed before deciding to go ahead with the surgery. You only get one chance at success. If you aren't ready to make the lifestyle changes, don't do it.

Other questions you may want to ask yourself:

1. Are the risks and costs worth the benefits?
2. What will I lose if I continue on my present path?
3. Can I honestly say that I have tried my best to lose weight without surgery?

Step 2: Discuss your thoughts and feelings about

the surgery with someone you trust. Be sure it is someone who will both listen to your point of view and offer you his or her own opinion. If possible, discuss your decision with several different people who have different viewpoints. It is tempting to just talk to people who will recommend the surgery, but do yourself a favor and talk to people who may be against the surgery as well.

Step 3: Do some research on your own. There is a wealth of information on the Internet and in books. Look at possible complications, the reality of the diet you will be on, and other risks. There are several different procedures available, and each involves risks specific to that procedure. It is important to take a hard and realistic look at the risks involved in the surgery. Candidates tend to discount the risks and emphasize the benefits at this point in the decision-making process.

Step 4: Look at success stories, and talk to as many people as you can that have had the surgery. If you don't know anyone, there are several chatrooms on this topic on the Internet. Millions of people have changed their lives for the better physically and mentally through bariatric surgery. Success can be about more than just weight loss. For example, did you know that bariatric surgery has been shown to lead to decreased comoribidites, and the Roux-en-y research shows that in more than 80 percent of cases, type II diabetes was resolved. What would you need to get out of it for surgery to be a success for you?

Step 5: Discuss your questions and concerns with the surgeon. The surgeon will be affiliated with a hospital-based program. You may request to speak to the dietitian, psychologist, and exercise physiologist with whom the surgeon works for even more details. Your insurance will probably dictate the facility and surgeon you will use for your surgery. Be sure to check out the surgeon, his or her track record with bariatric surgery, and any complaints that may have been filed against him or her.

Step 6: Take a look at your own weight loss history. Have you been able to reach your weight loss goals with traditional diets, only to then gain it back? If so, then losing weight is not necessarily the problem. Perhaps weight maintenance is your real challenge. Many of my clients tell me they have been unsuccessful at weight loss. In reality, they are very successful at weight loss because they have been able to lose substantial amounts of weight many times, but just need some good solid information on how to maintain that weight loss.

We have been programmed over the years to think of ourselves as either being on a diet or off a diet. Maintaining your weight after weight loss is something in between and requires a whole different mindset. The key to long-term maintenance is exercise. With exercise, you can maintain your goal weight while still enjoying some of your favorite foods. Take a look at your weight loss history. Is it weight loss or is it maintenance following weight loss that is the problem area for you?

If you have come to the conclusion that maintenance is your area of difficulty, then perhaps a healthy diet with the help of appropriate professionals can lead to long-term success. You may wish to consider consulting with a dietitian and a personal trainer or exercise physiologist. See a psychologist to help with those "excuses" we all give ourselves to stop exercising or to cheat on our diets.

Case Study

Jenny could not make a decision about the surgery. Her friends and family were concerned about the risks, but her doctor was recommending the surgery. She had already researched the procedure, spent countless hours thinking about it, and discussed all aspects of the surgery with people she trusted. She decided to make the Pros and Cons Graph, and she was shocked with the results.

She realized that her health would greatly improve with weight loss, and also that she would have to diet and exercise for the rest of her life even with the surgery. She decided to try a healthy diet and exercise plan one more time before having the surgery. All this became clear with the "Pros of not having surgery" box. Jenny said, "I just realized it would be better for me in the long run if I could do this thing without the surgery. I knew my health would improve with any weight loss at all, and it was time to get serious because this is about my health and quality of life. When I was really honest with myself, I realized I didn't want to hear that exercise was important even with the surgery. Once I accepted that exercise was required with or without the surgery, I just decided to give it another shot."

For Jenny, it took a couple of difficult months to really get into her new program, but after three months she had developed many new healthy habits. Both a personal trainer and dietitian were consulted during the initial weeks. She began exercising four times per week, and made many changes in her eating patterns. Jenny lost 36 pounds in three months, and has been steadily losing ever since.

Of course Jenny still had options. She was young and did not yet have any of the health problems associated with obesity. Many people are not this lucky.

The choice to have the surgery should be made with your doctors and people you trust. Some patients become glowing success stories, while others fall back into old habits and never realize their weight loss goals.

It may be worth one last try before taking the drastic step of bariatric surgery.

Step 7: Sit down with all of your information and do some honest soul searching. Bariatric surgery can change lives, but it is definitely not for everyone. Once you make a decision, let yourself live with it for a few weeks. With time, you will either feel more comfortable with your decision, or you will have that nagging feeling that you have not made the correct decision. With either choice, you owe it to yourself to take time in choosing whether or not to have the surgery.

How to Prepare Yourself Psychologically Before Surgery

There are many things you can do prior to surgery to prepare yourself, and all of these will increase your chances of success after surgery. Start the changes as far ahead of the surgery as possible. Shoot for at least 6 to 8 weeks before your scheduled surgery date.

The six main areas of preparation, which are all covered in more detail, are as follows:

1. Prepare your environment.
2. Prepare your support system.
3. Emphasize the activity rather than the food.
4. Learn to structure your eating pattern.
5. Control emotional eating/recreational eating.
6. Begin a consistent exercise routine.

WHY SHOULD I PREPARE BEFORE SURGERY?

Think of bariatric surgery as consisting of two entirely separate components: 1) the surgery itself—the creation of the pouch; and 2) the lifestyle changes. These lifestyle changes include stopping the emotional/recreational eating and maintaining a consistent exercise routine.

There seems to be an expectation that the surgery itself will force the lifestyle changes that must follow, but this is not the case. For the first 6 to 12 months or so, the surgery will make it easier to change your diet. This is called the "honeymoon period." It's easy to stay on the diet because you most likely won't be hungry and may get negative feedback if you do not follow the diet. For example, you may get sick or feel uncomfortable if you eat too much, eat the wrong foods, or do not chew enough, but after that initial period, it becomes mind over matter. The surgery will not force you to exercise or change your recreational or emotional eating habits. To successfully make all the necessary lifestyle changes, you will need to rely heavily on using your mind for adherence. We make lifestyle changes all the time, only to revert to old habits in three months, six months, maybe a year. To be successful with this surgery, you've got to make lifestyle changes for 30, 40, 50 years or more depending on your age. Your old habits must change for the rest of your life. Sound impossible? It is not, if you use the information contained in this book.

Lifestyle changes must last for life. This sounds simple, but how many times have you made lifestyle changes in the past, only to fall right back into those old eating patterns when you were bored, went through stress or changes at work, or went to a party and "blew it?" How many times have you lost weight, only to gain it all back? Did you go into the diet planning to gain it

Case Study

Margaret always had a sweet tooth. Thinking of her husband, she bought his favorite candy bars and ice cream every time she went grocery shopping. Coincidentally these were also her favorite candy bars and ice cream. When she was tired or bored, her resolve to stick to her diet seemed to disappear, and she often ate some of the treats that were in the house "for her husband."

There was always a full candy jar on her desk at work "for other people," but she was most often the one to indulge.

She seemed to plateau early in her weight loss. The nurse at the surgeon's office inquired about her eating habits. Margaret was confronted on the need to have her favorite foods in the house, and she conceded she was having great difficulty giving up her lifelong comfort foods.

Margaret agreed not to bring these items into the house again, and decided that her husband could get ice cream or candy bars himself if he so desired. The candy jar on her desk had to go, too. Through this experience, she began to understand the power of the mind in helping or hindering her in dietary adherence.

When Margaret was weighed the next month she had lost 15 pounds and had more control over her eating habits. She said, "I always had a really good excuse for keeping the food around, but now I understand these excuses keep me from achieving my goals."

back? Most people think, "If I can just take it off, I'll do everything I can to keep it off." Similarly, no one ever goes into bariatric surgery planning to gain the weight back, but it can happen. It is normal to fall off the wagon, but this time you can learn to use your mind to keep from going down that same road. The mind dictates your ability to stick with lifestyle changes, and this time it has to be for the rest of your life.

OUTDATED THINKING

Remember that lifestyle changes are separate from the surgery. Most people combine the two components in their minds, saying, "When I have the surgery, I will have to change my life." This is an example of outdated thinking when it comes to bariatric surgery. The old thinking is to wait for the surgery to start the lifestyle changes. The new thinking is to start the lifestyle changes as far ahead of the surgery as possible. This will give you more confidence and also give you a jump start on the long road ahead.

THE BEST ADVICE YOU WILL GET is to establish all of your healthy habits prior to surgery. The last piece of the puzzle is the surgery itself.

The best advice you will get is to establish all of your healthy habits prior to surgery. The last piece of the puzzle is the surgery itself. The most difficult part of the process is the lifestyle change, and if you master this before the surgery, you will do much better and have much less stress. By the time you add the final step of surgery, you are already on the road to better health. Patients who have prepared in this way report that it has been a positive experience.

Many people like to have "last meals" before the surgery. This is expected, but a much better use of your time is getting into all of the habits you must follow after the operation. Changing your lifestyle is difficult under the best circumstances, but after surgery when you may be tired, irritable, and sore from the procedure, it will be much more difficult.

BEHAVIORAL SURGERY

This is a whole new concept. If you have your tonsils removed it is up to the surgeon whether it is a successful surgery. When you have bariatric surgery, you will determine whether the surgery is a long-term success. With the lifestyle changes, almost any procedure will work. Without the lifestyle changes, no surgery will work long term. The lifestyle changes are always the most difficult part.

PREPARING YOUR HOME ENVIRONMENT

We all eat exactly the same thing. We eat "whatever's there." As I go through the years, I believe the environment, especially the home environment, is one of the most important aspects to weight maintenance. Your environment can make or break your success.

How many times have you said to yourself, "I didn't plan to eat the ice cream, but it was in the house and I had a moment of weakness?" Anyone who has ever attempted to change eating patterns can relate to this. The solution to this problem is to make sure you do not have foods in the house that will tempt you. It is imperative that you turn your home into a bariatric-friendly environment.

How do you make your home bariatric friendly? The key is to remove all trigger foods. Everyone has several foods that call to them from the refrigerator or the cabinet. It will be next to impossible to stay true to your bariatric diet if these foods remain in your home. After a hard day at the office or a personal crisis, it is very difficult to resist these foods. During a moment of weakness or hunger it is easy to eat the food, then immediately regret it. I hear this complaint from patients even years after surgery. Somehow those foods find their way back into the house, at about the same time willpower slips out the window. The first line of defense is to take all these foods out of your home. It is hard to do, but it is time to live your life without them.

WILLPOWER DOES NOT ALWAYS WORK

This is a difficult transition, but necessary if you are to achieve your weight loss goals. Trigger foods must be removed from the home. This is NOT an option. Trigger foods are the ones that we will eat if they are in the house. They are the foods we usually choose when we cheat. Everyone has a few of these. If they are present, it will be much more difficult to stick to your diet. When I see patients who are regaining weight, inevitably their trigger foods have crept back into the house, and they are eating "whatever's there." Compare it to a person who is trying to quit smoking. If there are cigarettes in the house, and others are smoking, it will be next to impossible to quit. How about the alcoholic who thinks he can meet his friends in a bar and just drink milk? Not very realistic, and he is putting himself in a situation where he will have to rely on sheer willpower. Willpower is not consistent, so the goal is to eliminate it as a variable in your weight loss. Set up your environment for success. Begin to create a bariatric friendly environment.

Become aware of roadblocks to success. Like a detective, scrutinize your environment, your home, your work environment, and your habits for obstacles. The goal is to completely take willpower out of the equation. When we rely on willpower, we are more likely to lose

Case Study

Dave knew before the surgery that his family was going to be trouble for him. Whenever he brought up the lifestyle changes he would have to make after surgery, his two teenage sons would say, "I hope you don't expect me to eat like you do."

He realized that if his family members were divided, it would be difficult for him to stick to the diet. Teenage boys tend to eat more and often bring junk food into the house. He knew the temptation at home was likely to be overwhelming for him. He also realized that his boys had learned some poor eating habits from him over the years, and he saw this as an opportunity to help them change these habits.

Dave called a family meeting and openly discussed his concerns and hopes for his sons. The boys listened and could see this was important to their father and likely to benefit them also. He made it clear that they would all benefit physically, and they would have more high-quality time with Dad because he would have the energy and mobility to engage in activities with them. He let them know that there was something to be gained for them as well. This was helpful as the boys did keep tempting foods out of the house. The last I heard, they took a bicycling vacation together and had a wonderful time.

the battle. Don't put yourself in a situation where you have to rely on willpower until you know you can handle it.

Be aware of the kinds of thoughts that entice us to bring certain foods into the house. If you think you must have sweets or some other nonbariatric food around for your family, then be certain to buy the items you don't like. Is it coincidence that when we bring treats into the house for "other people," these are our favorite treats as well? We'll even rationalize that somehow the family will suffer if they can't have your favorite trigger food in the house. What are the chances we can resist these foods when under stress, or when having a bad day, or having a craving? If you need an incentive, tell yourself your kids can live without cookies for a while and will probably learn some very healthy eating habits in the process.

When you reach your goal weight, you can do a little test. Try your trigger foods. If you are able to eat appropriate amounts, you may consider adding small amounts back into your diet. If you find you feel out of control with the foods, or are unable to regulate the amounts, then you may end up having to trade that trigger food for good health. Don't try this experiment until you've already reached your goal weight. A variation on this is one I prefer. If you love ice cream, for example, you can have it when you get to the goal. I recommend you plan it, enjoy it guilt free, have it once every two weeks, and go out to get a scoop. Don't bring it into your house because then it becomes very difficult to say no. There are no really bad foods, just foods you may have difficulty resisting.

CREATE A SAFE ZONE

Create a safe zone in your home by promising yourself not to bring in anything tempting or off your diet, regardless of the quality of the excuse. It is much more difficult to cheat if you have to leave your home to do it, and there are plenty of chances to talk yourself out of it on the way to the store. Imagine how much easier it will be to adhere to the dietary guidelines when you walk in your front door after work and can let down your guard. You won't have to worry about willpower or cheating. You don't need it because you are in a safe zone. In your safe zone are plenty of bariatric friendly foods and drinks, but no trigger foods. Remember, you do not want to rely on willpower to keep you on track, but rather an environment designed for bariatric success. This strategy boosts your chances of success, and is one of the most basic rules.

PREPARING YOUR SUPPORT SYSTEM

The people in your life will have an effect on your ability to stick with the lifestyle changes you must make. You will need to prepare them for changes they can expect, and to let them know the important role that they will play in your weight loss journey. Supportive family members will make it easier for you, and non-supportive family members can wreak havoc with your diet and your resolve to eat properly. Keep in mind that it is very difficult for family members during this

> **SUPPORTIVE FAMILY MEMBERS** will make it easier for you, and nonsupportive family members can wreak havoc with your diet and your resolve to eat properly.

process as well. I have a group just for the family members of patients, and no patients are allowed in. I hear things like "I feel uncomfortable eating in front of him," or "I remind her to take her vitamins and she snaps at me." It can be just as difficult being a family member to a patient as it is being the patient.

If you live with other people, it makes sense to

discuss with them the impending changes you will be making. I like to have whole families commit to using this as an opportunity to become healthier. Discuss any areas of concern with everyone living in the house as far ahead of the surgery as possible. If you approach your family with a coherent plan, they will be more receptive. Here are 11 questions to ask yourself:

1. How will meals change in the home?
2. What foods will and will not be available in the home? Discuss the concept of the safe zone.
3. How will the family benefit from you being healthier?
4. What can the family members do to help you be successful?
5. How should family members handle the situation if they decide to eat something they know will be tempting for you?
6. How will you handle having guests in the home?
7. How would the family like you to handle your new diet?
8. How will you deal with holidays and parties in the home?
9. Would your family like to use this as an opportunity to be healthier and more active themselves? If so, how can you all motivate and support each other?
10. Tell your family what to expect in the days and weeks after surgery. Explain the hospital stay and how you will need help completing some tasks for a while.
11. The radical dietary changes usually last about one year and then you are able to eat more normally, just with smaller portions. It often

helps to let the family know there is a light at the end of the tunnel.

Making sure that your family members are involved in the decision process will make it easier for everyone. If you are living alone, the changes will be a little easier for you. Often, family members are resistant to change because they are not the ones deciding to do this.

Make sure everyone in the family understands how this can benefit them, from losing weight themselves to doing more activities together. When you become healthier and lose weight, others will also reap the rewards.

RECREATIONAL AND EMOTIONAL EATING

It is very common to hear, "If I could just find out why I eat this way, it would be so easy to stop." Some people want to figure out why they eat for emotional reasons. The fact is, you don't need to know why in order to change. Even if you are able to get to the root

> **SOME PEOPLE WANT TO FIGURE OUT** why they eat for emotional reasons. The fact is, you don't need to know why in order to change.

of your emotional eating, that information will not usually automatically lead to change. It may be helpful to know why, and you may be very curious, but that knowledge is not of key importance to your weight loss. For most people, it makes sense to skip this quest, and proceed directly to the step of changing the habit. It is important to look at the emotions you experience when feeling out of control, but it may not be necessary to find the root of the problem in the past. It is not just how the habit started, but the repetition over many years that makes it hard to break.

Eating for emotional and recreational reasons is very common. I've spoken to patients from all over the world, and there are some things we all have in common regardless of our ethnicity, ancestry, or geographical location. Most of us grew up with food being central to family gatherings, holidays, even day-to-day life. Most of us were members of the "clean plate club," and we ate while being told to be thankful we weren't starving children in some faraway country. From the first time we fell off our bicycle and Mom gave us a cookie, we learned that food can compensate for a bad day, can be something to look forward to, can be very comforting. Even though this is a normal, and almost universal experience, if it is not reduced after surgery you may not have the long-term results you are seeking. Everyone does it to some extent, but giving in to that will make it very difficult to achieve lasting weight loss. You can prepare yourself to deal with those thoughts and situations so that food doesn't run your life.

Expect to always feel conflict about eating. Except for the first few months after surgery, you will probably want to go back to eating your favorite foods. If you expect the conflict, you can plan to deal with it and win the battle of recreational and emotional eating. In the beginning, most people will experience a decrease in hunger and cravings. This is called the "honeymoon period." It's easy to stick to the dietary regimen because you are simply not hungry.

	M	T	W	Th	F	Sat	Sun
Time							
Food							
Emotion before eating							
Unusual circum- stances							

Sample Emotional Eating Situations Form

The shock for many patients is that when the hunger returns, the cravings and thoughts of food do too. For a small percentage, they will never lose the cravings, and must battle the urges right after surgery. I have some patients that had the surgery four or five years ago, and they tell me it is still a daily struggle to remain true to a healthy diet. The hard truth is that if you use food for comfort or other emotional reasons, those thoughts and cravings will probably always be there. Research tells us that after surgery you will likely have six months to two years when your cravings and urges will be diminished, possibly even become dormant, but they will come back. Once the connections are established between food and emotions, they will not easily go away. They may diminish in intensity with time, but will likely be a part of your life for a very long time.

Before surgery, you can begin to experiment with eating only your planned meals and snacks, and when you crave food at other times, there are some things you can do. Start by keeping yourself busy, by taking yourself out of the situation, or by figuring out why you want to eat and finding another way to satisfy the need. Here is an example: You would normally eat to reduce anxiety, but instead of eating, try spending time on the phone with a friend or taking a hot bath. If you start to do this before the surgery, you will find several alternatives that work. This will give you confidence and prepare you for those same situations after surgery.

We eat because we are hungry and for a host of other reasons. Some common traditions and stressors that cause people to eat are family get-togethers and holidays or out of habit, anger, sadness, stress, and boredom. Or we create excuses for ourselves to make it acceptable, such as "It's Friday," "I'm celebrating," "I have to have wings because the game is on," or "I can't enjoy the movie without popcorn." You may not be hungry when you go to the family picnic, but when you get a familiar whiff of Aunt Betty's famous apple pie, you will want to eat it. This type of conflict will not go away, and it is the cause of much stress for the bariatric patient. You will gain confidence and control with experience, but expect to always have the cravings to some degree. One of my patients asked in reference to her love of food, "Will I ever get this monkey off my back?" The short answer is no. It will become a smaller monkey, and you will have much more control over it, but you should expect it to always be there to some extent. The monkey may become dormant, but it can come to life with stressful events or major changes in your life.

People have said to me, "When I don't want to eat during the honeymoon period, I'll just figure it out and never go back to my old eating habits." This way of thinking is completely unrealistic. Have you ever gone on a diet for six months, completely changed your habits, then at some point went right back to your old habits? This type of behavior is human nature. Just changing habits for a period of time does not guarantee they will become permanent. A better idea is to figure out what works for you right now to help you get past a craving or urge, and then use the same technique after the surgery. If you rely on hope, you may have a much more difficult time, and put the outcome of the surgery on the line.

✏️ ACTIVITY

Begin to look at all the situations in which you eat. Listing them is very helpful. Rate each one on a scale of 1 to 10 (with 10 being the most difficult to control).

Common reasons that show up on these lists are going out to dinner or a movie, holiday parties, sporting events, boredom, loneliness, sadness, celebration, or television viewing.

Try to set up your schedule and environment so they do not dictate whether or not you eat certain foods. Try not to put yourself in any situation you rated 6 through 10 until you know you are ready.

To use the Emotional Eating Situations Form, record the date, time of day, day of the week, the food you consumed, your emotion just before eating, and the circumstances at that time. After a few days, you will have a good idea of what emotions lead you to eat and you will understand how to intervene. For example, if you most often eat when bored, then perhaps starting various projects around the house, taking up a new hobby, or going to the movies will keep you from eating out of boredom. If you eat because you are lonely, then perhaps calling a friend or relative or visiting someone you haven't seen in awhile will be helpful.

Even though recreational eating is normal, it is something you should not do after surgery. Chances are you've been on many diets in the past if you are considering bariatric surgery, and you know how difficult it is to sustain strict dietary changes over time. Expect to always have conflict between the thoughts, "I really, really want to eat this," and "I know I shouldn't." Don't expect to magically not want to eat or be given some incredible willpower that you haven't had in the past. It is still possible to overindulge, and it is an all too common occurrence for people who have unrealistic expectations of the surgery.

Many people believe the surgery will prevent them from overeating, and they are both right and wrong. During the first few weeks after surgery, it will be almost impossible to overeat. You will be on a liquid diet, and food may not look very appetizing. It is when solid food is reintroduced into your diet that you must be careful. This usually occurs a few weeks after the surgery. Once you are able to eat again, you will probably crave your favorite foods. It will be a challenge to resist, just as it has been in the past. People tell me, "I won't eat the foods I'm not supposed to eat after surgery because it will make me sick." Unfortunately some people will try eating their favorite foods anyway, only to find they don't get sick.

Consider the person who is on a diet for diabetes and does not follow it. The consequences can be severe, but it does not stop people from cheating. The same is true of the surgery. Many patients think, "This will really stop me from overeating. This time I will have to do what I am supposed to do." Or, "Why would I eat the wrong foods when I risked my life for this surgery?" Or, "I'll get sick if I eat the wrong foods." This may sustain you for the short term, but don't count on it for the long term. The surgery will assist you, but it is still your decision whether you will cheat or whether you will stick with your bariatric diet. Like the person who is not following his or her prescribed diet for diabetes, people will cheat with this diet, too. The most powerful weapon to help you resist eating for life is not the pouch, but the mind.

REAL OR EMOTIONAL HUNGER?

For the new bariatric patient, you will most likely not feel true hunger for several months. It is important to eat as directed even when you might not be physically hungry. But for those starting these changes prior to surgery, or whose hunger has returned after surgery, it is important to distinguish between true hunger and head hunger.

True hunger, or physiological hunger, involves hunger pangs, stomach growling, or feeling weak or shaky from lack of food. This is the hunger that requires the response of eating. Over the years, many people lose the ability to recognize real hunger or differentiate between real and emotional hunger.

"Head hunger," or emotional hunger (also called psychological hunger or mouth hunger), must be controlled in order to be successful with long-term weight loss and maintenance. When you eat in response to a situation, like a holiday party or the smell of food cooking, or for emotional reasons, like stress or loneliness, you are responding to head hunger.

Ask yourself when you eat, "Is this true hunger or is this head hunger?" If the answer is head hunger, then it is time to change your environment, thoughts, activities, or situation. First take yourself out of the situation. Leave the kitchen, turn off the TV, or go outside and take a breath of fresh air. Take a short time-out to gain control, and then say something motivating to yourself, such as, "This is about my health, not food. I can do this."

Now that you have a realistic view of what to expect after surgery, imagine going to your first holiday party. Perhaps you had the operation four months prior and are feeling very confident. What will your strategy be? What will your escape plan be if you begin to feel overwhelmed? What will you say to people? Plan all of this ahead of time for your best chance of success. Remember, you will likely want to eat. Expect to have that conflict between wanting to eat and wanting to stick to the diet. Do not expect it to be easy for you. You may feel like you are on the outside looking in. It will get easier with time, but it will take multiple exposures to these types of situations to increase your confidence and your ability to stick to your plan.

BEGINNING THE FOOD EMPHASIS SHIFT

It is helpful to begin to think of food as fuel and your body as a work in progress. Every day will bring you closer to your goal as you lose a few more ounces and gain strength through exercise. Keep your eye on weight loss, improving health, and your long-term goals.

Food has been a "best friend" for some. If this is the case for you, there will be additional challenges. They don't call it "comfort food" for nothing. During times of stress, your thoughts may automatically turn to food, and you will have to override some pretty intense feelings in order to stick with your diet. I always suggest people write down when and why they eat. Are you really hungry? Or are you bored? Keep a list handy of alternatives to keep you busy, and call a friend if necessary. Get yourself away from the temptation, whatever it may be. My patients tell me they do well when they anticipate that changing habits will be difficult. Those that think it will be easy or automatic usually have a more difficult time.

Take steps to shift the emphasis from what you are eating to what you are doing. For example, instead of planning dinner out for Saturday night, think about the movie you will see or a trip to the beach to watch the moon rise. Most people dream of the exciting activities they will do when they lose weight. This is the time to think about and try those activities because it will give you power over eating and provide the motivation you need. Over time food will become secondary and will lose some of the hold it may have on your life. Don't wait until you are at your goal weight to begin enjoying those activities. Start now and it will be easier to stick to the diet because you are already enjoying yourself more.

✓ TO DO

Make a list of activities you can do instead of eating. When an urge to eat occurs, try one of the activities on your list. Keep the activities that work for you and discard those that don't. Another idea is to schedule your daily exercise during that time of day you are most likely to overindulge. Make sure your plan is realistic. It is not reasonable to expect to exercise every time you feel like eating. Some other positive activities could be to call a friend, take the dog for a walk, surf the Internet, have a glass of water, watch a

DON'T WAIT UNTIL YOU are at your goal weight to begin enjoying those activities you have always dreamed of doing once you lost weight. Start now and it will be easier to stick to the diet because you are already enjoying yourself more.

movie, read a book, get involved in a hobby or craft, and on occasion exercise. Of course you will still be able to eat, but shifting the emphasis to activity will help with the psychological transition.

STRUCTURED EATING PATTERN

Start some food changes a couple of months ahead of your surgery. Keep in mind that these lifestyle changes are entirely separate from the surgery, and everything you do ahead of surgery will lead to greater chances of long-term success. Start to structure your eating pattern. Have three healthy main meals and a couple of healthy planned snacks if you need them. Be prepared and shop ahead. If you take your healthy foods to work, it will go a long way to eliminate the desire for fast food and vending machine snacks. This will prepare you for life after surgery. Getting into the habit of always having healthy foods with you and avoiding the old habits will help make an easier transition. It is always better to rely on preplanning than on luck or chance.

You may also experiment with some of the bariatric foods you will be required to eat after surgery, and start teaching yourself how to chew each bite of food 25 to 30 times before swallowing. Begin training yourself to always have a bottle of water with you. Try to get in the habit of stopping drinking well before meal time and starting at least 30 minutes after you eat. You will be instructed to do this after the surgery, so trying to develop those new patterns in advance will only serve to help you later. These changes seem simple, but even retraining your automatic eating pattern requires concentration. It will take some time to become comfortable with not swallowing after just a few bites.

The Pre-surgery Psychological Evaluation

This chapter is meant to demystify the pre-surgery psychological evaluation. Surgery candidates often misunderstand the reason for the psychological evaluation and dread this appointment, thinking of it as a "roadblock," or "a hoop to jump through." The objective of the psychological evaluation is not to stop people from having the surgery, but to help people understand what they need to do as individuals to achieve long-term success. Altering the body will only get you so far. Long-term success requires learning to control the body and the mind. The ultimate goal of the evaluation is to help you succeed.

Problems occur in the psychological evaluation when people enter into it with an irrational fear of being told "no," or thinking of it as a "monster to get past." The psychologist's objective is to find out your individual strengths and challenges and to create a personalized strategy for your success. Honesty is the key element needed for the psychologist to achieve this goal. Any obstacle can be overcome with time, effort, and knowledge. In some instances, a patient has other health issues that must be addressed before a surgeon can perform a bariatric operation. So is the case with some mental issues. Oftentimes, these problems must be addressed before the surgery to increase the likelihood of a healthy and successful conclusion. But for some reason, people look at the physical state in a different light than the mental state.

The majority of surgeons and insurance companies require a psychological evaluation. The following are goals of the psychologist when evaluating patients for bariatric surgery:

1. Education of the patient about realities and risks of surgery (Can this person make an informed decision about the surgery?)
2. Identification of behaviors that may keep a person from losing weight or may lead to regaining
3. Helping the patient with personalized strategies
4. A written report created for insurance and/or the surgeon.

Here's what you can expect: There will be an interview lasting approximately 1 to 2 hours. These are usually conversational, and a lot less stressful than most people expect. Psychologists understand patients are a bit nervous, and will help you to feel comfortable with the process.

In addition to the interview, some psychologists will do testing. It may be extensive testing lasting several hours or there may be very little or none. If you are asked to take tests as part of your evaluation, try this approach. Be as honest and open as you can. Testing generally identifies personality traits and/or symptoms a person may be experiencing. You can ask for your scores and an explanation of what they mean when you meet with the psychologist for the interview, and it is all very interesting. Decisions are never based on testing alone, and there are no right or wrong answers. Test results are simply one aspect of information that assists the psychologist.

Why should I be honest? Patients with significant problems that were not quite ready for surgery sometimes say, "That's what I get for being honest. I should have lied." Imagine going to the cardiologist for your cardiac clearance and concealing chest pain in order to get that clearance for surgery. It does seem ridiculous, but people routinely do this in psychology. Lying in the psychological evaluation is only hurting yourself because the psychologist is looking for problems that would interfere with your success. People at times also believe decisions the psychologist makes are personal, but this is never the case. Showing up late for an appointment or "not hitting it off" would never be a reason to not recommend someone for surgery. Most people leave the psychologist's office feeling satisfied and armed with multiple personalized strategies for dealing with their own unique patterns and behaviors. The goal is always to get the person to the surgery.

What is the psychologist looking for? In general, your psychologist will be trying to understand your individual patterns concerning diet and exercise. We all have patterns, and we tend to fall into these patterns and pitfalls over and over again. Then, the psychologist may give you some personalized strategies. In order to do this, many different areas are explored.

First, we look at demographic and background information. You may be asked to fill out paperwork prior to your interview that will go into these details. Requested information will include how far you went in school, how many hours you work per week, and family living situation, including kids, spouse, and significant others. This also gives important information about your support system.

You will be asked about growing up, your brothers and sisters, anything that may be different than other kids, and if weight was an issue. You'll also be asked about any abuse that you may have gone through as a child. This will not impact your surgery, but if there is a history of abuse your psychologist will want to give you some additional information on problems that occasionally occur postoperatively.

You'll be asked about your habits concerning alcohol, cigarettes, cigars, and recreational drugs both now and in the past. The psychologist will probably talk to you about transfer of addiction during this phase of the discussion.

Stress is the enemy of lifestyle changes, so you will be asked about specific stressors you are experiencing at that time, as well as discussing how you deal with stress. The psychologist wants to know healthy activities in which you engage, such as reading, listening to music, doing crafts, or playing games.

You'll discuss emotional and recreational eating. Everyone does this to some extent, and you will discuss specifics during this section. The goal is to pinpoint the most difficult times for you and to give you strategies to deal with these situations when they occur in the future. Some examples are eating for comfort, fun, socializing, sadness, anxiety, or boredom.

Your motivation to have the surgery will be discussed. Why are you considering the surgery at this time? Is anyone pushing you to do this?

Your general understanding of multiple aspects of bariatric surgery will be discussed as well. You will talk in detail about your understanding of the procedure, both in surgery and how it works afterward; your understanding of the vitamin regimen and healthy diet

THE GOAL IS TO PINPOINT THE MOST DIFFICULT TIMES FOR YOU, and to give you strategies to deal with these situations when they occur in the future.

and the ramifications of discontinuing either; your understanding of the risks related to the surgery, both immediate and long term; your understanding of the importance of lifestyle changes, especially the exercise component; and your understanding of what happens when a person is nonadherent with the diet, exercise, vitamins, doctors' recommendations, follow-up bloodwork, and appointments.

You'll talk about your psychiatric history. This will include any inpatient treatment, outpatient treatment, and use of any medications, including antidepressants, antipsychotics, and antianxiety drugs. Mental illness is not a rule-out for bariatric surgery, but in general the psychologist will make sure you have a psychologist and/or psychiatrist that you see postoperatively on a regular basis so that you can be closely monitored for any increase in psychiatric symptoms. If you already have a psychologist or psychiatrist, the psychologist doing your evaluation will probably want to talk with him or her about how to help you after surgery because the area of bariatric psychology is very specialized, and most mental health practitioners are not aware of the potential problems facing patients after surgery. Be very forthcoming about this during your evaluation so the psychologist can set up that safety net for you. There is a higher incidence of suicide and depression after surgery, which makes this extremely important.

You'll talk about your diet and exercise history, and try to pinpoint what gets in the way of sticking with it long term. Everyone's pattern is different. No one has to watch their diet 24 hours per day. There will almost always be a particular place or a particular time when it is more likely you will eat something and then regret it. Thoughts and behaviors that get in the way of your goal to stick with the diet/exercise plan will be explored. Most patients find this very interesting.

At the end of the discussion you will be told the results and of any follow-up appointments or outside appointments that will be necessary.

The psychological evaluation is not just another appointment. It allows you to learn likely problems you will face after surgery and potential solutions. It's a good opportunity to ask questions too. It's educational and allows you to get to know the psychologist. Your program's psychologist will be an important part of your journey from early pre-surgery education through the hospital and through the support groups for years to come.

Self-Talk

A n important question that comes up when trying to adjust to lifestyle changes is, "How do we overcome a lifetime of recreational and emotional eating?" Part of the answer is in the concept of self-talk.

A very important key to your success following surgery is your ability to control your own self-talk. Self-talk is what goes on inside your head automatically. What you say to yourself will either put you in control of your life or give you a passive role in your own health and success after surgery. Controlling your self-talk is key to dietary and exercise adherence after surgery. Self-talk is discussed in many different contexts in this book, as follows:

- Using self-talk to increase motivation to exercise
- Using self-talk to control emotional eating
- Using self-talk for long-term weight maintenance.

Self-talk determines if you give in to eating the cheeseburger or say no and have the chicken breast. Self-talk determines if you skip your workout or go outside and walk for 30 minutes. Self-talk determines if you feel positive or negative about the surgery and your progress. Self-talk determines if you eat cookies because you are depressed or pick up the phone and call a friend instead. Self-talk plays a large part in life after bariatric surgery, and for many, it can ultimately determine success or failure.

Most people are unaware of the conversation that goes on inside their own heads all day, every day and are, therefore, unaware of the great effect it has on how they feel and act. In order to control your self-talk, you must first become aware of its existence. Let's look at some examples.

 ACTIVITY

Self-talk is not necessarily what we say out loud, but what we think and say to ourselves inside our heads. Test: Try saying something positive to yourself, and you will find that you instantly feel better than when you say something negative to yourself. For example, say, "This is going to be a good day." You will feel better than if you say, "Here comes another terrible day."

This internal dialogue takes place constantly, but most of us are not even aware of it and operate on "automatic." Think back to when you learned a new skill, such as using a computer, riding a bicycle, or

Tip

Think of your mind as a radio, and you control the radio stations. You can turn the channel from negative self-talk to a channel with positive self-talk. Remember, you have the ultimate control over your thoughts. They do not control you unless you allow them.

playing a sport. If you said to yourself, "This is fun. I know I can do it," chances are you did. If you said to yourself, "I'll never be able to do this," chances are you had difficulty. I talk to people who say, "I don't have self-talk. I just am the way I am." Everyone has self-talk and can learn to control it. It's just a matter of learning to recognize it.

Professional golfers and other athletes understand the power of the mind when it comes to success. There are psychologists who work exclusively with athletes to help them use these techniques to gain control of their behavior, reduce anxiety, increase confidence, and control the powerful messages of the mind. The messages you give yourself every day will have an impact on your ability to succeed in weight loss after surgery.

SELF-TALK: LISTENING TO THE EXCUSES

When it comes to diets, self-talk can determine success or failure. People start diets full of hope and motivation, but often that determination disappears by the third or fourth day. The culprit is usually self-defeating self-talk. How many times have you been on a diet and said to yourself, "I deserve a treat. I've been good all day." Before you know it, you've eaten something you did not plan to eat. Or how about when you say, "I'll just eat a little bit less tomorrow to make up for it." At that point, you have eaten too many calories for the day and may just decide to keep on going. The self-talk usually goes something like, "I've already blown it today, so I'll just start again tomorrow." The next day you find your motivation has greatly decreased and you may cheat again. By the following day you are off the diet completely. The next usual step is to say, "I'll just start again Monday," but when Monday arrives, your motivation has completely disappeared.

If this same person had said to herself, "If I exercise for 45 minutes today, THEN I can have that treat," or "I don't need that treat because this diet is about my feeling better and looking better," she might not have cheated.

A THEORY

Evolutionary psychologists have a theory. Human beings have been around for many thousands of years. For most of the history of our human existence, food was scarce and we learned to eat whenever possible. With the exception of the last few hundred years, people often did not know when they might be able to consume another meal. When it comes to exercise, conserving energy was a priority of our past because we needed energy to be available to fight, work, farm, or travel long distances. Things have changed radically. In the last few generations, calorie-dense, high-fat food has become abundant, and there is very little need in the lives of modern human beings to expend large amounts of energy. The result is that now we need to restrict our food intake and force ourselves to exercise to maintain a healthy weight.

If this theory makes sense, then you may agree with what happens next. Since "dieting" or "working out" are relatively new concepts for human beings, it is as if we are going against our own instincts, and something very interesting happens. Our minds begin to work against us, too. We actually become our own worst enemy. Our minds actually send us messages that give us long lists of really good reasons to stop dieting and exercising. Many psychologists believe we are "hard-wired" to say YES to food and NO to exercise. When we try to say no to food and yes to exercise, we are actually going against human nature. This is why self-talk is important. When it is time for a workout, our minds will begin to go through a list of possible reasons that allow us to skip that workout.

> **SINCE "DIETING" AND "WORKING OUT"** are relatively new concepts for human beings, it is as if we are going against our own instincts.

Almost everyone's mind works in this way. Call them "excuses" because that is the purpose they serve. With food, we will search for a good reason to consume the foods we know are not on our diets. Have you ever said to yourself, "Well, it is a special occasion. I'll just have a *little* bit of the cake." Or with exercise, one might say, "It is cold outside. I can't work out in the cold." Then tomorrow there is another reason. My experience with bariatric patients tells me that this internal dialogue of excuses will never go away.

Many times, the excuses may be true. The gym may be very expensive and it may be very cold outside. That's not why they are excuses. They are called excuses because we don't find a way around them. We don't exercise inside if it is cold. We let the excuses stop us from exercising. Accept that excuse-making is normal, natural, and part of life. Your challenge as a bariatric patient is to learn to ignore the excuses by overriding them through positive self-talk and behavioral strategies. Those who successfully lose the weight and keep it off are the ones who learn to recognize the excuses and decide to ignore them. You will want to listen to them. Learning to override them is one of the most important keys to long-term success.

One of my patients calls this the "devil on my shoulder." He says "I know what I'm supposed to do, but I have the devil on my shoulder telling me why I

> **THOSE WHO SUCCESSFULLY** lose the weight and keep it off are the ones who learn to recognize the excuses and decide to ignore them.

really don't have to. It's a constant struggle." When it comes to diet and exercise, there is a vast difference between knowing what to do and actually doing it. Use the power of the mind to tip the scales in your favor. You can win over the devil on your shoulder. Let's consider two different scenarios:

1. Mary gets out of bed and takes a shower. Afterward she looks in the mirror and says to herself, "You look disgusting. How could you ever

go out in public looking like this?" Her self-talk will now influence how she feels. She will likely leave for work feeling down, self-conscious, negative about the day, and not motivated to eat properly or exercise. As her day progresses and lunch approaches, she may make poor choices, asking herself, "What difference does it make anyway?" In the afternoon she has a big piece of her coworker's birthday cake, rationalizing, "This will be my last piece. I'm really going to hit the diet hard tomorrow." When she gets home she does not exercise, deciding, "It's been a hard day. I'll do it tomorrow." This cycle perpetuates itself as she feels even worse the next day.

2. Mary gets out of bed and takes a shower. Afterward she looks in the mirror and says to herself, "I am looking strong. I will take care of myself today, and tomorrow I will be even stronger and healthier. I'm a winner." Her self-talk will now influence how she feels. She will likely leave for work feeling better about herself and more motivated to eat properly and possibly exercise. When lunchtime approaches, she again uses positive self-talk by saying, "A healthy lunch will make me feel better, lose a little weight, and I'm worth it." She orders an appropriate lunch. Later, at the company birthday party, she says no thank-you to the cake because, "It's not worth the calories. I'd have to walk three miles to walk that off." When she gets home, she is tired from a hard day, but says to herself, "I can manage 30 minutes of walking. I'll feel better than if I skip it." This cycle perpetuates itself as she feels better the next day.

✓ TO DO

Make your long-term goals part of your own self-talk. If your choice is between eating the treat or not eating the treat, you will probably end up eating it. But if your choice is between eating the treat and working toward good health and you say to yourself, "I am working toward a healthier life, and I already feel better," you will have a better chance of saying no to the treat.

Remember how it works:

- **Positive self-talk** creates positive feelings, which in turn lead to positive behavior.
- **Negative self-talk** creates negative feelings, which in turn leads to negative behavior.

Again, wanting to cheat on a diet is normal, but you can greatly increase your control over eating and exercise if your self-talk motivates you and increases your determination.

Example: Picture yourself at the grocery store. Listen to your self-talk that goes something like this: "I know I'm on a diet, but that doesn't mean my kids (or spouse) should be deprived of their favorite cookies." This is one of many excellent excuses for bringing inappropriate foods into the home and is of course the first step toward cheating. This type of self-talk allows us to preplan our cheats by having these foods in the house. It also sets up our environment for diet disaster.

We all know that being on a diet is no fun and quickly becomes boring. We miss eating what we like, and we look for excuses to break our diets. Remember

Tip

Our excuses may be very clever. If you find yourself
skipping workouts or eating the wrong foods, ask
yourself why. Is this an excuse? What am I really doing?
What are the consequences if I eat this or if I skip
exercise?

that sticking to the prescribed diet after surgery is
much like sticking to any other diet, and you will
encounter the same temptations, negative self-talk,
and excuse-making that you have in the past. Even
though these thoughts are normal, they will eventually
keep you from your weight loss goals unless you learn
to control them. Whatever thoughts came between you
and success in the past will likely occur again. The
best defense is to expect it and be ready with a
strategy.

ACTIVITY—YOUR OWN SELF-TALK

1. **Spend several days tuning into your own
   self-talk.** Become aware of the rationalizations
   and justifications you give yourself to eat
   something that is not on your diet. Then decide
   you will not listen to this talk and that you intend
   to be successful.

2. **Make a list of positive phrases you can say
   to motivate yourself.** Every day will bring many
   opportunities to cheat on your diet, and having a
   few positive and realistic lines to get you through
   will be key to your success.
   Examples:
   "Food is not my friend."

"I have power over food; it does not own me."
"I'm feeling better than I have in years."

3. **Use your new positive self-talk when in stressful eating situations.** Keep the phrases that work, and discard those that don't.

4. **Expect to experience heightened anxiety when choosing not to eat in these eating situations.** Remember that anxiety is only a feeling. It can't hurt you. It will go away. Use your self-talk, and if all else fails remove yourself from the situation completely. An escape route is always an option.

5. **If anxiety is a problem, use a deep breathing technique.** Take five slow, deep breaths, and remind yourself why you had bariatric surgery.

6. **Utilize the "Thought-Stopping" technique.** This is a strategy for stopping a negative or self-defeating thought in its tracks. The second you realize you are having one of those thoughts, do two things:
   A.   Picture a large, red stop sign in your mind.
   B.   Say "STOP" to yourself.
   This will help you clear your mind so you may proceed with replacing the thought with one that will assist you in meeting your goals. An alternative to the stop sign is to wear a rubber band around your wrist and snap it gently when you find your thoughts are out of control. Either one will work until it becomes second nature for you.

7. Use the "What If" technique. This self-talk technique has been useful for people who eat for comfort. When we try to stop eating a particular comfort food, or stop eating in specific situations, people may feel anxious, keyed-up, on edge. They think the only way to make the feeling go away is to eat the food. Instead, ask yourself, "What if I don't eat it?" The answer is "I'll feel uncomfortable, anxious." Then ask yourself, "What if I feel uncomfortable and anxious?" The answer is, "Nothing will happen. Being uncomfortable or anxious cannot hurt me." Then ask yourself, "What else can I do to help me reduce this anxiety?" The "What if" technique helps us see that the anxiety that comes from not eating may be uncomfortable, nothing more.

CHANGING NEGATIVE SELF-TALK TO MORE REALISTIC TALK

At times, our negative self-talk becomes completely unrealistic. During these times, it is useful to know how to change that negative thought to a more realistic one. An example of negative or destructive self-talk would be, "I've had a terrible day. What would it hurt if I just had some of my old comfort foods for dinner? I'm miserable without my favorite foods. Maybe I shouldn't have had the surgery." Obviously the person in this example is on his way to cheating. He can avert diet disaster by listening to his own self-talk, recognizing how it makes him feel, and deciding to make changes. He may use a Thought-Stopping Technique, and then replace that negative thought with one more likely to benefit his health and help him meet his weight loss goals.

An example of more realistic and positive self-talk would be, "I'm progressing daily, I can walk two miles now, and I couldn't walk out the door three months ago. I'm feeling good, and that's all that matters. I can do this."

✓ TO DO

1. Tune into self-talk.
2. Recognize excuses.
3. Use the Thought-Stopping technique.
4. Override excuses.
5. Replace excuses with realistic self-talk.
6. Use the "What If" technique.

MOTIVATIONAL VISUALS

A variation of self-talk is having a motivating picture that you can use to say "no" in familiar eating situations.

✓ TO DO

Use your mind as a photo album that shows the future. You will open that photo album in your mind when needed. The album should contain photos of yourself in your future. You are at your goal weight. What are you doing? What are you wearing? Who are you with? You are happy, healthy, and enjoying yourself.

Use your mental photo album any time. Your mental photo album provides a visual of the best aspects of your goals and will assist in keeping you on track.

** Any decision you make concerning eating and/or exercise will impact your ability to reach your goal or your ability to stay at your goal. Always ask yourself "will this get me closer to my goal weight or keep me from the goal weight."

Case Study

Karen described herself as a "sneak eater." She said she always ate appropriately when people were watching, but once she was home alone she ate all the wrong foods. For her, the challenge was to continue to make wise food choices even when people were not looking. Since she was unable to always eat with other people, she began by making some rules for eating. She started eating only at the table, only at regular meal times, and only with planned foods. She removed all of her trigger foods from the house. When she found herself thinking of eating in secret, she used a visualization technique. She pictured the one person she least wanted to catch her sneak eating. In this case it was her mother. She pictured her mother standing next to her, arms crossed, looking disapprovingly at her. She told me that picture in her mind was just what she needed to stop. Once she was able to refrain for two weeks, she said it got much easier for her. She says she still has the urge now and then, and at times even gives into it, but credits using her visualization technique to finally helping her control a lifelong problem.

The 3-Point Plan

You can inoculate yourself for stressful situations full of conflict and emotions and give yourself a better chance of success by following this strategy. Before you go into any situation that is likely to be difficult or in which you previously ate whatever you wanted, devise a plan. Think about three things that make up our 3-point plan:

1. What you say to yourself
2. What you say to others
3. What you do.

Rehearse your plan mentally several times, and when you go to the event you will be much less likely to do something regretful. This strategy has worked for many people I have counseled, and it can work for you.

Let's consider a hypothetical family gathering for which you need to devise your 3-point plan (what you say to yourself, what you say to others, and what you will do). How will you get through the evening without eating too much or eating the wrong foods?

1. WHAT YOU SAY TO YOURSELF

Some people say to themselves, "This is about my health, and I'm a healthy and different person now." Some say, "Food got me into this situation, and I'm not going to let it beat me." Or "This is about my family, not the food." Or "I'm worth it." With practice, you will find the phrases that get you through the tough spots. I advise everyone to begin experimentation before surgery with self-talk, and start a list of phrases that work for you. Say your motivating phrases when you feel like cheating or when you feel anxiety because you are not eating something you want.

Now that you have a couple of phrases of positive self-talk to help during your family gathering, the next step is to think of what to say to other people.

2. WHAT YOU SAY TO OTHERS

Some people like to be open in conversation about the surgery, and others feel it is a private matter. The most important thing is to be aware of how you are most comfortable and plan your strategy with that in mind.

When Uncle Charlie pressures you to try his famous potato salad, you will need to be prepared with a response. Perhaps you can say, "That sure looks good. Will you make it for me again in six months when I can try a bite?" The keys are not to give in to pressure and to have a response that allows you to stay in control. Some patients tell me they eat all the wrong foods at gatherings because they do not wish to alienate anyone.

3. WHAT YOU DO

The third part of the strategy is to plan what you will do when in the situation. This step involves the behavioral logistics of the party. For example, you may plan to avoid the hors d'oeuvres table, keep a glass of water in your hand, and have any conversations far away from the food. When the dinner arrives, you may plan to have three bites of the meat and two of the vegetable, and leave the table if it becomes overwhelming for you. The possibilities are endless, but the point is to have a workable plan prior to the party, and it should be a comfortable strategy.

MENTAL REHEARSAL

Whatever your plan is, it is helpful to rehearse mentally before you arrive. This will help you stick to it. Some basic tips to mental rehearsal are to sit in a quiet place and picture the scene in your mind. Be sure to use all your senses with this technique. The more vivid the scene, the better. Think of what you will hear, smell, see, taste, and how the air will feel over your skin. You will most likely experience an increased sense of control and find your experience unfolds closer to your ideal plan than if you had not used mental rehearsal. This is a popular technique with professional athletes because it works.

Hint

Savor your food and enjoy it. It is really only a matter of quantity. This way you will feel less deprived.

Even if mental rehearsal is not used, be sure to think about what you will say to yourself, what you plan to do, and what you will say to others prior to arrival.

Planning ahead in this manner offers a much better chance of success than simply hoping for the best or relying on others to keep you from eating. This proactive planning will put you in control and boost your confidence as well.

Now, you can apply your 3-point plan to various situations you will experience as a bariatric patient. Let's take a look at several of these situations.

YOU'VE BEEN INVITED TO A PARTY

Going to a party for the first time after surgery can be both exciting and overwhelming. This may be the first chance for your friends to see you after having lost a couple of sizes. Remember to have your 3-point plan prepared and mentally rehearsed prior to arrival at the party—what you will say to yourself, what you will say to others, and what you will do. For many, this is the first real test after surgery, and it can be highly anticipated, dreaded, or something in between.

Your weight loss will likely be the subject of much conversation. You have reason to be proud, but not everyone is comfortable being the center of attention. You have worked hard and gone through many changes in order to be where you are. If possible, enjoy the attention.

It is normal to feel as though others are watching you as you eat at the party. They are probably curious as to what you are able to eat. You may enjoy the attention, or you may feel uncomfortable. Plan your strategy with the idea that people will be

Tips

1. Once during the evening, go to the hors d'oeuvres table. Take a few items and nibble. Don't worry about throwing some away if you take too much. If this is difficult for you, consider eating before the party and commit to just talking and sipping your drink. For some, it may be easier to avoid the food altogether than to eat a preplanned amount.
2. Keep a glass of water, iced tea, or other flavored water or noncaloric drink in your hand for sipping throughout the party.
3. Try to steer your conversations away from food. Remember to concentrate on the activity rather than the food.
4. You can discuss your weight loss or not, but the choice is yours. It is acceptable to ask that the subject be changed if you wish. On the other hand, it may be motivating for you to discuss it with people. It is entirely up to you.
5. Have a plan for how you will leave the party if you begin to feel overwhelmed. Always have an escape route. Some plan ahead to spend only two hours.

curious. On the other hand, chances are they are not paying quite as much attention as you think they are.

Try to relax by using some of your relaxation techniques, such as deep breathing or calming self-talk, if anxiety is a problem for you. If you prepared yourself properly, you will begin to feel comfortable in a short period of time.

When you leave, having followed your plan, pat yourself on the back. It is not easy going into a situation where you previously may have consumed food and/or alcohol. You are on your way!

YOUR FIRST DINNER OUT IN A RESTAURANT

This is a big test for the bariatric patient who has recently had surgery. Your first decision will be what to say to the waiter. Some people like to mention they have just had surgery and will need their food prepared according to specific guidelines. Others are a bit more private and would rather just order their food without butter or oil and with sauces on the side. Either way, you can order from the appetizer menu and most likely be full, or you can order from the dinner menu, eat your regular portion, and take the rest home.

Some of my patients like to split dinners in restaurants. You will find the method that suits you with time, but it is your choice whether or not to disclose that you have had surgery. It is not necessary to tell a waiter why you order a particular way, unless it makes you feel more comfortable.

A common fear is, "What if the food gets stuck or I have a problem at the restaurant?" The first bite often determines how the rest of the meal will be tolerated. Be sure to take your time and chew your food thoroughly. Anxiety about eating in a restaurant can make it difficult to swallow, so remember to relax and take slow deep breaths if you're feeling anxious. You may also request a table near the restroom. The host will probably be grateful for a chance to seat someone there voluntarily. If the worst does happen, it is not the end of the world. Simply get up from the table and walk to the restroom. Chances are you will be fine. Welcome back to the world of restaurants.

THE HOLIDAYS ARE HERE!

It starts on Thanksgiving and ends on January 1. This is the time of year when we traditionally let go and enjoy large amounts of food without worrying about

Tips

1. Choose a restaurant where you can order your meal prepared to your specifications. You may ask for your food without butter or oil or with sauces and dressings on the side.
2. Keep your mind on the activity of socializing rather than on the food itself.
3. Have your 3-point plan prepared and mentally rehearsed.
4. Ask to take the leftovers home with you, or better yet, ask for a "to-go" container as soon as your food arrives. Place most of the meal in the container before you begin eating. This strategy also assists with the "clean plate" compulsion. In this way, you can be a member of the clean plate club without overeating.
5. Concentrate on the people you are with and the interesting conversation rather than just the food itself.
6. Begin to notice the sounds, sights, and smells in the restaurant. Take it all in. There is so much more to the experience than just the food.
7. Enjoy the food, too! The only difference is quantity. Savor it and enjoy it.
8. Some restaurants will allow bariatric patients to order from the children's menu, but be careful what you get. These meals are often high in fat.

calories. It is a part of our upbringing and culture. Everyone else is doing it, and we do not want to feel deprived. Along with all the cheer and gift giving is food—and lots of it. How do you keep from gaining weight or significantly slowing down your weight loss during this time period? By planning.

Realize it is human nature to let down your guard during the holidays. The psychological connections are so strong, it is difficult to maintain healthy habits, but not impossible. I always find an influx of patients coming to support groups in mid-January. The usual complaint is they fell off the wagon in November and have been eating much more than recommended through the New Year. Many have gained weight and stopped exercising. Planning is the key to surviving the holidays with minimal disruption in your bariatric diet and exercise plan. It is possible to maintain your weight or even lose a bit.

✓ TO DO

1. **Just after Halloween, sit down and really think about the holidays.** Ask yourself what foods you are most interested in during this time and what foods you would be willing to give up for health. Make a list of foods you choose to keep. These are usually the ones that have the most meaning or are your favorites. Also list the ones you are willing to give up. These are usually the filler foods or snacks that are present during the holidays but that you could live without. Keep the lists handy, as you will need them when Thanksgiving approaches.

2. **Next, set up some rules while you have a level head unclouded by holiday excitement.** An example might be to allow yourself an alcoholic beverage once per week and choose the specific day. Another example might be to try your mother's sweet potato casserole, but only three or four bites on the holiday itself. The idea is to have what you really love, without adding all the other mindless calories. You can do this and still maintain your dietary regimen.

Problem

"My pouch is bigger, and I can eat more, so I am overeating."

Solution

Shift your thoughts from "I must eat until I am full," to "I must eat only until I am no longer hungry." Remember it is not necessary to fill the pouch to capacity.

3. **Commit to following your diet as though it were not the holidays with the exception of the special foods on your holiday list.**

4. **Commit to continuing and even increasing your exercise regimen during the holidays.** Many are tempted to stop during this period, but exercise can limit the damage done by the extra food. Life gets more hectic during the holidays, but there is always time for exercise. Remember the benefits of added energy and stress reduction that exercise provides. It is very difficult to restart an exercise program once you let it go. Exercise should remain constant throughout the holidays.

5. **Ask your family for assistance.** Share the lists with them and ask that they not bring these foods to your home.

6. **Consider having holiday meals at another person's home instead of having the family to your house that first year.** Don't put yourself in too many situations where willpower dictates your choices and your health.

Tip

Begin to think in terms of quality versus quantity. You will be able to eat many of your favorite foods eventually, but in much smaller amounts. You are not deprived, just eating smaller quantities.

If all else fails, go to the section of this book called Emergency First Aid. I often get frantic phone calls from patients who cannot seem to get back on track. With preplanning and sensible rules, you will do well during this time of year.

YOU CAN STILL COOK FOR THE FAMILY WHILE ON THIS DIET

Another situation that will need preplanning is how to cook for the family and for yourself. It is always a good idea to discuss this with your family prior to surgery so everyone will know what to expect. There is no universal way to handle this, and it will depend on the dynamics of your family and what you are able to handle.

One of the easiest ways to prepare dinner for everyone is to prepare a protein, such as fish or hamburger. It can be prepared in many healthy ways, and you simply eat less than everyone else. Include a vegetable and other side dish for the family, and you are ready. This method allows you to eat the same foods as the rest of your family. It is healthy for the family and is easier on you because you will not have to resist some forbidden food they may be having. It is important for some people to not feel like an outsider at mealtimes because that may be a stimulus for cheating.

On the other hand, a few people have told me they prefer having separate meals because it emphasizes that they are on a very special program. If you fall into this category, you may decide to cook completely separate meals for the rest of your family. If you follow this course, do not be tempted to eat the food you're cooking for others. You may only be able to do this after several months on the diet and after developing a certain indifference to food and confidence in your self control.

WHEN YOU ARE NOT THE COOK IN THE HOUSE

What happens when you are expected to eat what someone else is cooking for you? You may decide that you will cook for yourself or may discuss with the family the idea of everyone eating healthier. The important point is that you don't put someone else in charge of your adherence to the diet. If the only way you can have the required foods is to cook them yourself, this may be your best bet. Another option is to find a local restaurant that will prepare food to your specifications.

CAN FUN FOODS BE A PART OF THIS DIET?

YES, absolutely. After an initial period on a liquid diet and a step-up to pureed foods for a short time, you will be able to eat solid foods. Your program's dietitian or your surgeon will provide you with a list of things you are allowed to eat. While sticking to the diet you will lose weight, but there are countless exciting ways to cook the proteins that comprise the main portion of your daily food intake. I have seen bariatric-friendly dips, skewered and grilled chicken, and hors d'oeuvres that look delicious. Be creative. Just because you are on a restricted diet does not mean it has to be boring and repetitive. Also, keep your eyes open for new cookbooks for bariatric patients.

I HAVE SEEN BARIATRIC-FRIENDLY dips, skewered and grilled chicken, and hors d'oeuvres that look delicious. Be creative. Just because you are on a restricted diet does not mean it has to be boring and repetitive.

TEENAGERS AND BARIATRIC SURGERY

Teenagers face a unique set of challenges on the road to success. One of the biggest is the total comprehension of lifestyle changes they must make for the rest of their lives. It is difficult for a teen to imagine being 20 or 30 years old, let alone 70 or 80. Because of this, teens may not understand, or take seriously, the long-term ramifications of stopping a vitamin regimen or doing annual bloodwork. The benefits of the surgery can be worth it, but for less mature patients it can be quite a challenge. Full understanding of what lies ahead is critical.

Here are a few tips. If you are a teenager, it will be tempting to have your parents cook and shop for you. Consider the idea that it should not be your parent's responsibility. A much better idea is to plan for yourself by putting the items you need on the family shopping list. Food preparation after surgery is a very time-consuming activity, and this is YOUR lifestyle change. It involves planning ahead, shopping, cooking, cutting foods into small pieces, packing lunches, and can take many hours per week. You have been found to be mature and responsible if you have been cleared for this

Case Study

Shauna was always an introvert. She had a few friends, but kept mostly to herself. When I saw her for the presurgery evaluation it was clear this was a person who knew who she was. She was more mature than the average 16-year-old girl and was intelligent with a good sense of humor. After surgery, she lost close to 200 pounds and was very excited. I saw her again about two years later, and she appeared to be depressed. She told me she was one of the "in-crowd" now. She had dates for the first time, all the latest styles in clothes, and felt "normal" for the first time in her life. She also told me she was unhappy. She had not been exercising or taking her vitamins and had been drinking too much alcohol. We talked for a while, and it became clear that she had stopped seeing herself through her own eyes and started measuring herself according to what others thought. Before the surgery she did not respect the so-called "in-crowd." After the surgery, she became part of the in-crowd and no longer respected herself. But being popular was not the problem. The problem was that Shauna gave others power over her sense of self. It can be highly seductive for teens to feel like everyone else, even "popular," for perhaps the first time in their lives. Emotions are hard to predict after surgery, and changes can be life altering. Shauna decided to put herself on a "social diet," much like a food diet, and to take back control of her health and her future. She decided to make a place in her life for social activities and friends, but not to the exclusion of health-related activities like exercise. When I saw her a few months later, she said she felt better and that just taking back control had made a difference.

surgery, so this is an opportunity to really take charge of your own health.

Since you will eventually move out of your parent's house and have to take care of yourself, it makes sense to take responsibility from the beginning. Think of it as a part-time job that will require much preplanning, preparation, and energy. I advise all of my patients to take personal responsibility for their own lifestyle changes, especially teenagers. This way, when you do move out of the house, it will be a much easier transition.

The biggest obstacle will be peer pressure and wanting to feel like your friends. Your friends might not have to worry about exercise, vitamins, support groups, or watching their diets. They may push you to forget about these things, and you may want to feel like they do.

SNACKING

Snacking has been associated with regaining weight after surgery. It is possible to fill up the tiny pouch many more times during the day than your dietitian will recommend. Even though snacking is considered healthy for some before surgery, afterward it can cause problems. Be sure to eat only the snacks recommended by your dietitian. Some patients report snacking up to 15 times per day. This will translate into less weight loss overall and possible regain of weight down the line.

I knew of a patient whose story illustrates this rule. Before surgery she used to eat an extra-large pizza every night, which is not all that uncommon. After surgery, she did well for about six months. At that point she was able to eat without getting sick, and she started to eat pizza again. At nine months she was back to eating an extra-large pizza every day. She would cut it into hundreds of tiny pieces and eat it throughout the day. Her weight loss quickly reached a plateau and then she began to regain. She had relied on the surgery to stop her, but ultimately it was up to her, not the surgery, to stop this behavior.

Beginning a Consistent Exercise Program

There are many psychological tips and strategies to exercise adherence. When working with bariatric clients, I encourage them to start their exercise program well before having the surgery. Getting into the exercise habit prior to surgery increases your confidence and sets the stage for success.

Exercise is a very important component to a patient's life after bariatric surgery. Exercise during weight loss will help you stay more toned, feel more energetic, and become stronger. It can burn more calories and assist in the weight loss itself. But the real surprise to many people is that exercise is even more important after you reach your goal weight. Successful weight maintenance is a product of proper eating and continued exercise.

I have heard horror stories of people gaining weight back, either because they reverted to previous eating habits or because they did not continue to exercise. When I see someone for the presurgery psychological evaluation, I always discuss the importance of lifelong adherence to an exercise program.

Start by setting aside some time, at least five days per week, and get in the habit of exercising on those days. It is fine to just walk for 5 to 10 minutes if that is all you can manage at this time or to stretch and use upper body weights for a few minutes. The most important aspect of preparation is to get into the habit of scheduled exercise and to overcome the excuses used to skip workouts. Consistency is the key. With time you will be able to walk farther or work out for longer periods of time. To succeed, you must get into the habit of exercising no matter what else is going on in your life.

I often hear people say, "I lost the weight and never exercised." It is possible to do that because the decreased food intake causes most of the weight to come off. However, it is very difficult to KEEP the weight off without exercise. People who choose this course are at a very high risk of being unsuccessful in the long run.

If you need another motivation to exercise, try this: Exercise is one of the best proven stress reducers. New research shows that exercise can work about as well as an antidepressant—without the side effects—if done on a regular basis. Also, since stress and depression are potent triggers to eat for many people, you can see how exercise can become a very important and powerful tool for weight loss and maintenance. Exercise will give you the quality of life

Tip

Would you describe yourself as a stubborn person? I have found that self-labeled stubborn people do well after surgery if they take a couple of steps:

1. Tell others not to push you or to remind you of what you should be doing. Stubborn people have a tendency to do the opposite.

2. Tell yourself that you will not let anyone or anything get in the way of your goal. Tell yourself that nothing will keep you from exercise, and no one will convince you to eat something you should not. Tap into that stubbornness and use it to your advantage.

that you are seeking. If you picture yourself walking all day at the theme park without getting tired, it's not just weight loss that gets you there, it is the exercise.

Exercise is for life. This is a harsh reality, but a fact of life nonetheless. Everyone knows someone who is thin, eats whatever he or she wants to eat, and never gains weight. It is unfair, but you are likely on the other end of the spectrum. Once you realize that it isn't fair, but it is reality, you are in a position to begin making lasting changes. There are two ways to look at this: Either, "It's not fair. I don't want to. I'm too busy," or the better way, which is, "It is not too big a price to pay to finally take this weight off and keep it off." For whatever reason, once a person gains weight, then loses weight, exercise is required to keep it off for life. We don't have a magic pill, but for now exercise and surgery is as close as we can come.

You may be exercising now. If so, you are way ahead of the game. You may have tried to start exercise programs numerous times but have been unable to stick with it, or perhaps you have never really exercised. Whatever your situation, this section will give you tips and techniques to get you going and keep you on track.

EXERCISE AND SELF-TALK

We all enjoy exercise immediately AFTER the workout. The problem occurs just before the workout when we start making excuses not to do it. How many times have you skipped a workout after saying to yourself, "I'm too tired," or "It's too late," or "It looks like it's going to rain," or "I don't have to exercise on vacation." The list of possible excuses is endless. This self-talk allows us to skip the workout, but deep down inside we know the truth. The next day we are feeling a bit sluggish and start with the excuses again. Often we end up saying, "I'll just start again tomorrow. I'll really get into it again tomorrow." Of course, tomorrow never comes.

Thoughts such as these are absolutely normal. Everyone battles these excuses daily, including surgeons, athletes, psychologists, and dietitians. If you want to be successful with exercise maintenance, it is time to learn to ignore and override these excuses. It is not possible to stop exercising and keep all the weight off for life.

Consider the people who go on regular diet and exercise plans and lose substantial amounts of weight. Then they stop both exercise and healthy eating when they reach their goal. The weight returns, but they complain that the diet did not work. Actually the diet did work, but they did not make permanent lifestyle changes; rather, they made the changes only until they reached the goal. If these people had simply continued to exercise, they would have likely kept most of the weight off. This type of thinking illustrates normal human responses to lifestyle changes. We tend to drift back into our old habits. It is exactly the same after bariatric surgery. Use your motivational techniques to avoid this trap. When you get to the maintenance stage, focus on your program, your habits, and avoidance of those excuses.

In order to motivate yourself, it helps to discover your long-range goals. These goals will become part of your positive self-talk and that will help motivate you to exercise even when you do not feel like it. Here are some tips to finding your internal motivation:

1. Perhaps you are experiencing a deterioration in health. Say to yourself one of the following: "I will exercise today because my health is the most important concern in my life right now;" "I can't

What are my excuses?

To find your own excuses, make a list of all the reasons you do not exercise, have skipped a workout in the past, or have ever quit an exercise program. Now look for ways around those reasons. For example, if you are exhausted after work, then try working out early in the morning. If the gym is closed when you want to work out, then buy some home equipment or just do some walking in your neighborhood. It is normal to have reasons not to exercise, but do not let those excuses keep you from your goal of losing weight and keeping it off for life.

wait to feel good again;" or "If I exercise today, I am one step closer to my goal of good health and feeling good again."

2. If your real motivation is to look good, then say: "Each time I exercise, I get closer to my goal of looking great and wearing that bathing suit." You may wish to look at a picture of yourself when you were once at the weight you now hope to achieve, or use a magazine picture of your fantasy goal.

3. If your goal is to have energy to get involved in activities, then say, "A little work today will help me be able to hike in the woods with energy, or swim in the ocean, or shop at the mall without shortness of breath."

4. If your goal is to be able to keep up with the kids, then say, "I'm doing this for the kids. They are worth it, and they will love having an active parent again."

5. If your goal is to turn back the clock in general, then perhaps try, "I can't wait to feel good again, and exercise will get me there." Or "My spouse isn't going to recognize the new me."

Your motivation might include several of the above, or something else completely individual to you.

It is not uncommon for a patient to tell me that he or she just does not like exercise. He or she is often under the mistaken belief that everyone who exercises likes it. Sure, some people love exercise, but the vast majority of us do it because of the benefits. It is similar to brushing your teeth or taking a shower. When we are very young, we are taught these habits. Most of us resisted them. We might have pretended to take a shower or just dampened our toothbrush. Eventually, we came to appreciate the benefits of toothbrushing and bathing. Now, we would not dream of skipping our shower or not brushing our teeth. We don't do it because we enjoy it; we do it because we have to in order to be clean. I know of no one who looks forward to brushing their teeth. We

> **ADDING ANY HABIT TO YOUR LIFE** is difficult, but one requiring time and effort, such as exercise, will take many years to become automatic, like brushing your teeth.

learned these skills as children, and we do not question them now. Exercise will eventually become like that, but it will take years to get there. Can you imagine someone saying, "I'm just not a toothbrushing kind of person," or "I used to be a toothbrusher, but it was boring, and I was changing jobs so I was really busy and didn't have time to brush," or "My arm was sore so I stopped." The excuses may be true, but we would never let that stop us from brushing our teeth.

These excuses seem ridiculous when applied to brushing our teeth, but are routinely used to avoid exercise. Adding any habit to your life is difficult, but one requiring time and effort, such as exercise, will take many years to become automatic like brushing your teeth. Our minds actually work against us by providing a list of excuses so we do not have to exercise. Learn to recognize and override those excuses. Millions of people exercise every day, not because they like it and not because they are motivated but for one reason—to keep weight off.

STARTING THE EXERCISE PROGRAM

Starting an exercise program can be both exciting and frustrating. It takes approximately six months to a year for exercise to become a habit. Some people will learn to love exercise and some never will. For the first few weeks you will be more tired than usual, but if you stick with it, you will notice an increase in energy. Before long you will feel stronger and sleep better. Exercise is a natural antidepressant and is good for your heart. It is a stress reducer, decreases anger and hostility, and gives you a sense of control over your life. It may be one of the greatest things you can do for yourself, but it takes work.

One of the most elusive aspects of exercise adherence is making it a priority. As a bariatric patient, your health has to be the priority, and

EXERCISE is a natural antidepressant and is good for your heart. It is a stress reducer, decreases anger and hostility, and gives you a sense of control over your life. It may be one of the greatest things you can do for yourself, but it takes work.

exercise is an integral part of your health. It may feel awkward asking your spouse to watch the kids so you can go walking or postponing making dinner so you can go to the gym, but it is necessary. Keep in mind that your insurance company, surgeon, and hospital staff are all on your team and working toward your good health, but exercise is completely under your control. They are your cheerleaders and are there to help if you need it.

The idea of putting yourself first may be foreign and uncomfortable and may be followed by guilt, especially if you have always been the caretaker of the family. Push yourself through those feelings, and they will diminish with time. Remember that if you take care of yourself, you will be better able to take care of your family.

I have talked to many people who were able to change their eating habits, but who never became consistent with exercise. They did not think it was necessary because they were losing weight. Eventually they began to gain weight back. Exercise is one of the most important components to long-term weight loss maintenance. There is no way around that fact. It is not fair, but it is reality. Once you understand the necessity of adding exercise, you are halfway there.

HOW MUCH SHOULD I EXERCISE?

The professionals in your bariatric surgery program will likely vary on this answer. Most will tell you to gradually increase to 3 to 5 times per week or more and for at least 30 to 45 minutes per workout. If you can make it part of your daily routine, that is even better. Aerobic exercise is excellent, and adding free weights or equipment is a good supplement. Walking is a great way to begin, and it is inexpensive, simple to do, can be done from home, and can be as easy or intense as you choose. Whatever your choice of exercise, remember to discuss it with your doctor.

Start small. If all you can do is walk for two minutes, then that is a good place to start. Perhaps by the next week you will be able to walk 3 or 4 minutes. Think of an exercise continuum where you are at one end (at the beginning) and Olympic athletes are at the other end. You may never be an Olympian, but at least now you are on that same continuum.

If you are in a wheelchair, do simple upper body stretching or use two-pound weights to begin working on the arms. Perhaps you buy a DVD of upper body aerobics or get into a pool and use the resistance of the water. Try to look at what you can do, not what you can't. With time, you will be able to do much more.

START SMALL. If all you can do is walk for two minutes, then that is a good place to start.

The most important part in the beginning is just getting into the habit of working out. It seems simple, but this is one of the most difficult phases of exercise. Battle that negative self-talk and ignore the excuses. Making these excuses is normal—and all people that exercise experience them—but they are what stands between you and your goal.

Here is a helpful strategy. If you skip a workout for any reason, say to yourself, "I choose not to exercise." This helps to keep the right perspective on exercise and assists in taking responsibility for skipping workouts rather than using some external factor as the reason. It is easy to blame skipping workouts on having "no time," but realistically there is time; we just choose to use it for something other than exercise. Make a commitment to yourself that if there is not enough time to exercise, something else will have to go, not the exercise. Perhaps the dog gets a bath tomorrow, or maybe the bills get paid later in the evening. There is always time for exercise if you make it a priority.

DO I HAVE TO SPEND A LOT OF MONEY TO JOIN A GYM?

You absolutely do not have to spend a lot of money by joining a gym. Going to the gym is not for everyone. You can exercise from your home or around your neighborhood and still achieve your weight loss and weight maintenance goals. On the other hand, some people enjoy the camaraderie, easy access to personal trainers, access to top-of-the-line equipment, and available support. It is an individual decision, and some have both a gym membership and a home exercise program.

If you are not a gym person, don't choose the gym for your exercise program. You will be setting yourself up for failure. Most bariatric patients I know already have a gym membership that they never use. The thinking may have been "If I spend money on a gym membership, I'll be motivated to use it." It hardly ever works out. If you are not a gym person, you'll look for a reason not to go.

WHAT EXERCISES SHOULD I CHOOSE?

Boredom is the enemy in an exercise program. Try activities you are interested in or ones that you may have enjoyed in your past. Choose between walking, rollerblading, swimming, walking in a pool, joining a gym, bicycling, hiking, water aerobics, tennis, golf without a cart, using free weights, mall walking, and many others. Some people choose several activities and alternate depending on their mood. Expect exercise to be boring most of the time, but you are not doing it for entertainment. You are doing it for your health and your future. On the other hand, some people really find they enjoy exercising and look forward to it. Others set goals and achieve amazing things they thought would never be possible. I have met people that have completed marathons and triathlons and climbed mountains. They found an inner athlete. Perhaps there is one in you.

ARE THERE ALTERNATIVES TO THE 30- TO 40-MINUTE WORKOUT?

Sure. An interesting variation is to do three or four 10-minute workouts during the day. It may be easier to fit in 10 minutes on the treadmill four times a day than to set aside one large block of time. Taking this route requires extraordinary determination because you must motivate yourself

AN INTERESTING VARIATION is to do three or four 10-minute workouts during the day. It may be easier to fit in 10 minutes on the treadmill four times a day than to set aside one larger block of time.

to exercise several times each day. It is also helpful to purchase a pedometer to wear all day. By the time you reach your goal weight, you should be able to accumulate at least 10,000 steps per day.

Either way, you need to choose to exercise. Along with the long workout, or several short ones, you can also add small opportunities to burn calories throughout the day. Start parking farther away from your office building, grocery store, or mall. Take short, energizing strolls throughout your workday. Walk the dog a bit farther than usual. It all adds up. These can't be considered enough for your exercise requirements, but they do help.

QUESTIONS

There are several other questions to ask yourself when making your exercise choice.

1. **How much will it cost to buy the equipment?**
   Be realistic about what is within your budget. You do not need to spend a lot of money or join a gym. Exercising from home is a good choice, and walking is inexpensive. All you need is a good pair of walking shoes.

2. **Will I have to travel to do the exercise?**
   Consider how accessible your choice will be. If you join a gym, there is an extra step to exercising as you must drive to the gym.

3. **Is there too much preparation time involved in doing my everyday workout?** Do you have to prepare a large amount of equipment? Is there a time commitment for maintenance of equipment?

4. **Is it something I think I will enjoy or have enjoyed in the past?**

5. **Do I need an exercise buddy to motivate me?** If you need a partner, then activities where you will be accountable for missing a workout would be a good choice for you. Perhaps joining a gym, joining a team, or having appointments with buddies or a personal trainer would be beneficial.

6. **Am I interested in this activity?** If it doesn't interest you, it will be next to impossible to sustain the exercise routine. Just because your friend likes water aerobics does not necessarily mean it will be a good choice for you.

7. **What will my backup exercise choice be if it is raining or my partner is unavailable?** Always have an exercise video, free weights, or some other type of physical activity planned for when nature interferes with Plan A.

8. **Will I actually do the exercise I choose or will I feel too self-conscious?** Be realistic. I have been told by many patients that they will not go to the gym until they have lost 50 pounds. If this describes you, then perhaps purchasing a stationary bicycle or doing exercises at home is a better choice on a temporary basis.

9. **If you have special needs or are not able to exercise due to pain or mobility, you will need to consult an exercise physiologist.** Most hospital programs have one on staff, and together you can creatively design an exercise program that will meet

your needs. Some of my patients in wheelchairs do aerobic videos designed just for them. These videos emphasize upper body movements, and I have been told that they are enjoyable. As you lose weight and hopefully gain mobility, your exercise program will evolve.

KEEP AN EXERCISE LOG

An exercise log is a helpful tool for long-term success. It is motivating to see your progress and reinforcing to add another workout to the list. Another advantage to logging your workouts is the ability to look for trends. What time of day feels best to you for exercise? How many days per week of exercise works best for you? How does your workout feel if you missed a few days in a row? I know people who use their logs to track their feelings, their weight, and even major life events. Log books keep you honest. It motivates as well if you have to write "no workout" on skipped days.

Exercise Log

Date:

Time:

Exercise:

Rating:

Comments:

Case Study

George had bypass surgery four years ago. At 410 pounds he had diabetes, high blood pressure, sleep apnea, and joint pain. He reached his lowest weight of 210 pounds about one year later. George was ecstatic. His diabetes and sleep apnea had disappeared, blood pressure was in the normal range, he took fewer medications, and his joint pain had significantly reduced.

He came to a group recently having regained more than 80 pounds. He had been told by the surgeon to exercise, but he couldn't make himself do it. He would exercise once, and then stop for a week or two. He was aware of the repercussions of not exercising. He refused to go to therapy to work on the thoughts that keep him from exercising. He stated, "I just don't like exercise. I can't do it. I don't want to do it."

George disregarded his doctor's advice and never began to exercise. Without it, the prognosis is poor that he will ever lose the weight or stop regaining. On his last visit, it was determined that his blood pressure was increasing and joint pain was returning.

Here is another trick. If you skip a workout you must write the reason in the log book. "No time" is not an option since there is always time to find at least 20 minutes. It may be at 5:00 am, or during lunch, or while catching the news in the evening, but in most circumstances, there will be an opportunity to fit at least a short workout into your schedule. You must be very honest with yourself. If you have 30 minutes to watch TV, you have time to exercise. Challenge yourself to be as healthy as you have the potential to be.

All the research confirms that self-monitoring tends to help people stick to a diet/exercise routine. I like the exercise log for an additional reason; it serves as an early trip-wire. If you are writing down your workouts every day, and writing down "no workout" on days when you skip, you will be able to see when you are slacking off. Because of our human tendency to lie to ourselves about working out, we might not see that we've stopped until it's too late. Research shows that when a person stops exercising for a full week, it is generally six months until they get started again. If you can see your logbook everyday it will tell you if you need to put on those shoes and exercise. Don't let it go an entire week or you may be in trouble. Use a logbook as your early trip-wire.

In your logbook, you will indicate the activity you participated in, the time you spent doing it, and the speed or pace, if appropriate. It is helpful to devise a rating system, such as a scale from 1 to 5, to rate your overall experience. When you achieve a 5, take note of the factors that contributed to such a great workout so you can recreate them.

There are several types of logs from which to choose. There are exercise logs available for purchase at most major book stores, and they come in many different sizes and price ranges. Some excellent software is also available for tracking workouts. The advantage to the software is the ease of entering data. All of your exercises, routes, and preferences can be entered beforehand, and keeping up with your log involves just a few keystrokes. If you are computer savvy, there are some free exercise logs on the Internet. You simply join a free site, are given a password, and can log your workouts online. With both the Internet and software, you can generate charts and graphs of your progress, and most can track weight loss as well. There are programs available for your smart

Tip

Think of yourself as an athlete. If you are exercising at all, you are an athlete. You may be a beginner, but you are an athlete.

phone too, making it very easy to enter information no matter where you happen to be.

MOTIVATION TO EXERCISE

Let's face it. If motivating yourself to exercise was easy, we would all be out there daily. Motivation is inconsistent and often elusive. This section will address issues related to the difficulty most people experience in beginning and sustaining an exercise program.

When given the choice to exercise or not exercise, most people will choose not to exercise. Realistically, it is an effort. It's not much fun, and we would rather not do it at all. But that is not really the choice anymore. The real issue here is your health. Exercise is just a means to an end.

Motivation is not a trait. You are not naturally an unmotivated person. Chances are you are well motivated in many areas of your life. The challenge is to motivate yourself specifically for exercise.

Motivational tips. Since exercise motivation is a problem for most people, here are some tips that may help when you need it. Motivation can be high one week and low the next. Increasing motivation will likely be an issue for life. Listed are some motivational strategies for exercise. Experiment and see what works best for you.

1. **Play some upbeat music as you get dressed to exercise.**

2. **Buy some magazines that feature your sport or activity.** There are magazines for walking, running, bicycling, surfing, bodybuilding, hiking, mountain biking, swimming, triathlon, and many others. Just seeing them sitting on your coffee table can help motivate you. You do not have to be a professional athlete to learn valuable information about your sport from these publications, and they can really get you excited about being involved.

3. **Join a group.** There are walking groups, swimming groups, groups that do only calisthenics, roller hockey teams, softball leagues, jazzercise, water aerobics clubs, and many others. The advantage of these is having other people counting on you to show up. If you know self-motivation is a problem, perhaps knowing others are expecting you will help. Playing on a team is a good idea if you enjoy the sport, and you would benefit from having an ongoing appointment for exercise.

4. **Along those same lines, it sometimes helps to make a pact with an exercise buddy.** Making a commitment to be there for your buddy can help you stay consistent with your program. However, if your exercise buddy cancels you must still exercise. The trap is that you may end up putting someone else in charge of your exercise program. Make a commitment that you

will work out with your buddy, but if they are unavailable, you will still exercise. The buddy is the icing on the cake.

5. **Purchase a new piece of equipment or new workout clothes.**

6. **Enter an event, such as a three-mile walk for charity.** Listings are located on the Internet or in the newspaper. Get some others involved, and make it a group activity. Give yourself several months to work up to the distance.

7. **Set goals and rewards for sticking to your program.**

8. **Increase the rhythm of your breathing slightly.** With each inhalation say the word "energy."

9. **Start a pre-exercise routine that gets you in the mood to exercise.** Olympic athletes use this technique. You might include stretching, repeating a motivating word to yourself, and listening to a favorite song as you dress for the workout.

10. **Use distractions, such as a portable radio, CD player, MP3 player, GPS speed/distance system, or talking pedometer.**

11. **Save an interesting mental activity for your workout, such as planning your wish list for the holidays, planning your next vacation, or planning your child's next birthday party.**

12. **Imagery is a powerful psychological technique.** It involves using your mind to create a vivid mental picture. Use energizing pictures like a locomotive or a tiger ready to pounce. These images will help you feel more energetic and ready to exercise. You may wish to imagine your body full of white energy. Whatever image is energizing to you is just right.

13. **While exercising, you can use imagery to help you through your workout.** For example, while walking or jogging you may imagine you are being pulled by a rope or pushed by a giant hand. Imagine you are in an exotic location or crossing a finish line in front of crowds of screaming fans. The possibilities are endless.

14. **Pay ahead.** If you want to eat something extra, don't say to yourself, "I'll exercise more tomorrow." Instead, pay ahead. Exercise more today, and then decide if you still want to eat that something extra.

15. **Use time management and organizational techniques and prioritize your schedule.** This will help to eliminate obstacles in your lifestyle change and give you more time for exercise.

16. **If you find yourself getting bored, change something.** Try a new exercise, vary your routine or route, or buy a new piece of equipment or clothing.

17. **Grandma's rule.** Remember when Grandma would tell you, "You can't have dessert until you eat your vegetables?" You probably did eat the brussel sprouts so you could have dessert. You can use this technique for exercise, too. Try, "I won't have dinner until I finish my three-mile walk," or "I won't surf the Internet until I go to the gym." The technique works. If you have a treadmill or exercise bike, use the first half hour of your favorite television program on the equipment, then sit down to enjoy the rest of the show. It's very difficult to get back up off the couch to exercise.

18. **Hire a personal trainer.** Personal trainers are very motivating. Some even come to your house. Be sure to check their qualifications thoroughly.

19. **Use advancing technology.** There are computer programs that sync with exercise equipment. You can race the computer on your exercise bike on a simulated race course. These programs even make it more difficult when riding uphill. Technology will only increase, and the cost will decrease over time. Try the Wii Fit™ for another alternative to traditional exercise routines.

THE 5-MINUTE RULE

There will be times when you find it almost impossible to motivate yourself to exercise. The 5-Minute Rule was designed to use in these "motivational emergencies." It is based on the reality that just getting started is the most difficult part.

Let's say you just can't motivate yourself today. Here's how the 5-Minute Rule works. Tell yourself you only have to exercise for five minutes. Go ahead and put on your workout clothes and get started. If after five minutes you just can't go on for any reason, even if it's just because you are not in the mood, you may quit. At least you know you gave it the old college try. You will probably feel more motivated the next day, rather than less motivated if you had completely skipped the workout. Sometimes magic happens. Most find that nine out of ten times you will choose to keep on exercising when your five minutes are up, because the hardest part is getting dressed and starting in the first place. Either way, you win. You end up doing the workout, or you feel like you at least tried.

GOAL SETTING

A little known and highly motivational technique is goal setting. Goals challenge you. They are extremely motivating, and it feels great when you achieve them. A goal or a series of goals is necessary to help direct

CAN'T SEEM TO GET MOTIVATED? Tell yourself you only have to exercise for five minutes. Go ahead and put on your workout clothes and get started. If after five minutes you just can't go on for any reason...you may quit. At least you know you gave it the old college try.

your exercise, to keep you focused, and to keep you motivated.

There are two types of goals: long-term goals and short-term goals.

Long-term goals. These are the BIG goals. It may be to walk five miles, do a triathlon, play hockey, or ski for five hours straight. It is anything that may have seemed out of reach to you before.

Short-term goals. These are the STEPS needed to achieve the long-term goal. Often called "bite-sized goals," short-term goals should be:

1. *Realistic.* You may be able to only walk 100 yards at first. Do not set your sights too high. If you haven't exercised in 20 years, give yourself a break. You can always add time, speed, or distance as you meet each short-term goal.

2. *Measurable.* You should be able to measure your progress in miles, time, number of days per week you work out, etc.

3. *Moderately difficult.* Research shows people work harder for goals that are not too hard and not too easy. Set the bar for yourself somewhere in the middle where you will be challenged but not too much.

4. *Specific.* Write out your goals. State how many days per week you intend to do what you have chosen. Depending on what activity you choose, you should also indicate the time you will take to do it, or the distance you will go. If you plan to walk two miles four times a week, you are likely to work harder to achieve

that goal. Some people even make up a contract for themselves that specifically states the rewards.

TO DO

Write down your long-term goal and then the short-term goals you will use to achieve it. Plan your week each Sunday evening and attempt to adhere to your plan.

Example: My Goals and Plan

My long-term goal is to walk a 5K race (3.1 miles). I will choose a race that is five months from now.

1. My short-term goal is to walk 1/2 mile per day (about 10-15 minutes), four days per week for the first two weeks (Monday, Wednesday, Friday, and Saturday).

2. At Week 3, I will extend my walk to 3/4 of a mile (about 15 to 20 minutes), and by six weeks I will be walking one mile per day (about 20–30 minutes), four days per week.

3. At Week 8, I walk 1 to 1.5 miles per day (about 30–40 minutes), and two miles (about 40–50 minutes) by Week 10.

4. At Week 14, I will walk three miles (about 60 minutes) twice per week.

5. By Week 20, I will enter a 5K walk for charity.

REWARDS

Achieving goals is much more motivating if you attach a reward. If you can't motivate yourself for a health reason, how about a new DVD or new clothes?

There are two types of rewards: internal and external.

Internal rewards. These rewards are the physical and psychological benefits we get from doing the activity. They include a sense of accomplishment, pride, energy, strength, enjoyment, and feeling better. These are potentially present every time we exercise.

External rewards. These rewards are treats we promise ourselves for meeting our goal. It should be something you desire enough to work toward and something you would not ordinarily purchase for yourself. Some new clothes, a new CD, the T-shirt you get at the 5K, a mini-vacation, or a power tool are examples. Of course your pocketbook will dictate the types of rewards you plan, but the key is you only receive the reward if you achieve your goal. Another type of external reward is more intangible, such as a vacation day from work to use as you please. Whatever you choose, it can serve as a great motivator when you really need one.

You may choose a goal such as the Presidential Physical Fitness Award. It is available for adults, and information is on the Internet at www.fitness.gov. There are patches, certificates, and other motivational rewards for meeting requirements in 100 different sports and activities, such as walking, bicycling, and aerobics. There is even a category for doing a combination of different activities.

It takes about six months to a full year for exercise to become a habit. The external rewards will

IT TAKES SIX MONTHS TO A YEAR for exercise to become a habit. The external rewards will help get you to that point. After it becomes a habit, it will be more difficult to skip your workout, and the internal rewards may be enough to sustain your motivation.

help get you to that point. After it becomes a habit, it will be more difficult to skip your workout, and the internal rewards may be enough to sustain your motivation. You can reintroduce rewards into your program any time that you need them.

A large percentage of people quit their exercise programs. Do not let that be an option for you. Flip that switch in your mind from "I hope I have time to workout" to "Nothing will keep me from working out."

To be successful in sticking to your exercise program, remember these tips:
1. List your long-term and short-term goals, and attach rewards to your effort.
2. Log all workouts. Your log will be an early trip-wire for developing problems
3. Use the motivational tips.
4. Prioritize exercise in your life. Your weight and health depend on it.
5. Do not expect instant results.
6. Give it a chance. It takes about six months to a year to become a habit.

7. Learn to ignore that negative self-talk and turn it into positive self-talk.
8. Remember that exercise works to prevent weight regain in the maintenance stage of weight loss.

Some general pitfalls to avoid:

1. **Don't count what you're doing during your day as exercise.** I often hear from my patients, "I have a very active job. I'll count that," or "I walked up the stairs today. I'll count that," or "I parked farther away at the grocery store. I'll count that." Although these are helpful, they are simply not enough. The exercise needed postoperatively will always be over and above what you do during the normal day. Anything "extra" is helpful, but not sufficient.

2. **"I didn't see results with exercise, so I quit."** The results of exercise after bariatric surgery are generally invisible. You will keep the weight off, feel better, have more energy, but the results will be invisible.

3. **"I'm just not an exercise person."** Very few people are. Remember you don't need to be motivated or love exercise to do it. I know some people that absolutely despise it, but do it simply for weight maintenance.

4. **"I'm just too busy."** The body doesn't know the difference between a good excuse and no excuse. It won't matter if you are working 20-hour days at work, saving the world, or just sitting on the couch flipping channels…the result will be the same.

5. **"I'm not motivated."** Somewhere along the line we decided to put exercise into the "optional" column, when in reality it is in the "mandatory" column. Why do we go to work? Because we love it? Or because we want the paycheck? Why do we pay the IRS? Because we like the IRS? Or because we want to avoid the consequences of not paying? Why do we stop at red lights? Because we have extra time on our hands? Or because we don't want the ticket? We do all these things because we want the results and to avoid the negative consequences. We don't do them because we are necessarily motivated. Exercise is exactly the same. Take it out of the "optional" column, and place it into your "mandatory" column, and it will be easier to do. No more "trying" to exercise, say "I will exercise because I want to keep the weight off."

6. **"If I liked exercise like he does I'd be out there every day too."** The truth is he probably doesn't like it either, but does it for his own reasons. I'm inviting you to join millions of us, surgery or not, who exercise every day and do not like it. Welcome to the club.

7. **"No time."** Sure you have the time. If we had to do a computer game for 30 minutes per day to keep weight off we'd find that time. Sometimes it is at 4:30am. This isn't for everyone, but if you have a seriously full schedule, consider exercising early in the morning. I know many teachers or people with two or three jobs who choose morning exercise. It's not crowded, there are no beepers, no phone calls, no kids, and best of all it's done by the time you go to work, there's no need to worry about it again

until tomorrow. If you plan to do it after your second job, and arrive home tired, how likely is it you'll be able to follow through? If you'd like to try this, start by getting up half an hour earlier and doing 15 to 20 minutes of exercise. Just increase this over time.

8. **"I travel. I can't exercise."** A common thought is, "Exercise is more difficult for me to fit into my schedule now, therefore I can't." The solution is to have a Plan A and a Plan B. Plan A is your daily routine, when you are at home and everything is

Case Study

Beth traveled for a living, spending half of each month on the road. She had a banding procedure and had not met her weight loss goals. She followed the diet and exercised while at home, but never mastered planning ahead for travel. While on the road she ate in restaurants and did not exercise. Since she had an expense account for meals, it was difficult not to get the most out of it. In the group meetings, people gave her suggestions, but she never tried any of them. Eventually she stopped going to group meetings. Almost three years after her surgery, Beth decided to get more serious, and she went back to her group meeting. We discussed her creating a Plan B for travel, and we all helped her iron out the details. She would bring protein shakes with her and have those for breakfast rather than the French toast she had been choosing. She purchased a fold-up stair stepper that she kept in her suitcase and got up early to workout in her hotel room while watching the news. She started to lose weight again, which reinforced her motivation to succeed. She is not yet to her goal, but because she addressed the problem, she is now much closer.

predictable. Plan B may be for a vacation, work/travel, or the weekend. This is when you may plan to have a treadmill brought to your room in your hotel, or bring a rubber band resistance set to the hotel and get up a half an hour earlier to work in your exercise. Perhaps you plan to walk a half hour in the airport with your carry-on baggage after you pass through security. Any plan will work as long as you proactively address the problem before you go and come up with a realistic solution.

Exercise is usually the biggest challenge for most patients. Use these tips to your advantage. Don't strive for perfection. If 9 times out of 10 you can do your workout you'll be just fine. Develop the voice within yourself that says "I need to exercise today," and be accountable to yourself. Call your program's psychologist and go to groups if you find you have stopped.

Behavior Modification

Most everyone has heard the term *behavior modification*, but few truly understand its application to diet and exercise. In this section, you will learn specific strategies to help you stay consistent and on track with your lifestyle change goals. These tips will greatly increase your ability to make the necessary changes and help your transition to a healthier lifestyle.

Behavior modification is a set of small changes you can make that will assist you in learning your new habits. Habits are very difficult to change, and certain aspects of your environment and some of your normal behaviors will make it even more difficult. Behavior modification is based on the idea that powerful psychological connections between certain cues and eating are established over time. Examples are watching football and eating chicken wings or coming home from work and immediately making a sandwich. These habits are normal for most of us but must be changed in order to be successful with weight loss. Because the psychological connections tend to be very strong, there is a tendency to fall back into old habits. These behavior modification techniques will make it easier to start new, healthier habits.

Habits in general are formed by repeating the action over time. New habits are formed in much the same way. Starting new habits is more difficult because it also involves resisting an old habit. This transition is stressful for most people. Refer to the section on stress reduction to help with this change. When we resist an old comfortable habit, we will usually feel some anxiety. This does not mean that you must go back to the old habit to feel better. A better alternative is to learn behavior modification techniques and cope with anxiety in a healthy way so you can progress with your lifestyle change goals.

When you attempt to change any habit, there will initially be anxiety. Learn to cope with the anxiety by using relaxation and deep breathing techniques. Power through the transition period and you will be successful at changing the habits that make weight loss difficult.

The first step to starting behavior modification is to figure out your particular triggers, cues, emotions, and situations that lead to emotional, recreational, or habitual eating.

✓ TO DO

All that is required for this activity is paper and a pen. For the next seven days, you will record everything you eat, what was going on at the time, and your emotions.

This activity can be completed before the surgery or after the surgery if you find yourself drifting back into old eating habits.

Spend one week recording everything you eat. Write down the time of day, what you ate, what was going on at the time, and the predominant emotion just before you ate (lonely, tired, stressed, happy, etc.). Write down everything, even if it seems insignificant. The payoff comes when you have a week or more worth of data to examine.

When you have at least seven days of information, sit down and look for patterns:

1. Are there one or more predominant emotions that seem to lead to eating?

2. Is there a particular time of day or night that appears to be more troublesome for you?

3. Is there a particular place that triggers eating?

4. Is there an activity that triggers eating, such as watching TV?

5. Is the presence of particular foods a trigger?

6. Is a particular day more of a problem than others?

7. What about automatic or mindless eating, such as snacking or nibbling while cooking?

8. Try to distinguish between internal cues (e.g., sadness, excitement) vs. external cues (e.g., television commercials or the scent of food cooking).

Once you have this information, you are in a much better position to begin making changes. When you understand the places, emotions, foods, time of day, and other patterns that lead you to eat, you can commit to avoiding these triggers, changing your environment or recreational pattern, and looking for alternatives. Change the routines that always lead to eating. The key is to become aware of the triggers, and then to make planned, alternative choices to avoid the trigger or change the situation.

As you begin to change these connections between cues and food, they will lose some of their power over you. They will always be there to some extent, but you will learn to take control of the situation rather than let the situation control you.

SPECIFIC BEHAVIOR MODIFICATION STRATEGIES FOR WEIGHT LOSS

Begin to look at your home and work environment like a detective. What specific behaviors, habits, or aspects of your environment interfere with making lasting lifestyle changes? These cues can be eliminated or at least greatly diminished. Use the data you have from your food log to pinpoint the key problems and then try the following strategies:

1. **Eat only as advised by your bariatric doctor.** Usually this will be three meals per day. Try not to allow yourself to snack between recommended meals while making this transition. If you must, make it a bariatric-friendly snack.

2. **Eat very slowly and place your eating utensil on the plate between bites.** As a bariatric patient, you will be advised to chew

your food at least 25 times, so this in and of itself will slow you down.

3. **Do not engage in other activities during mealtime.** Concentrate only on eating. Avoid reading, watching television, or too much conversation. This time is about eating only.

4. **It is most important to eat in a specific place.** Choose a room where you will do all of your eating, and promise yourself not to eat anywhere else. If possible, eat in the same chair. Do not eat while driving or doing other activities as you will quickly lose track of the amount you have consumed. It is important not to establish a connection between driving and eating.

5. **Stay out of the kitchen except when absolutely necessary.** Think of the kitchen as closed. Keep the kitchen light off so the room is not so inviting, and try to take alternate routes that don't lead you past it if possible. Make sure food is stored only in your kitchen.

6. **Use small plates, bowls, and utensils.**

7. **Do not keep leftovers on the table to invite additional nibbling after you finish.** Instead, get up from the table immediately and do something else. It may be helpful to store leftovers in the refrigerator or freezer before your meal so you will not be tempted to eat more later. This technique requires you to go through several time-consuming steps to get to the food, and at any of those steps it is possible to stop.

8. **Keep food out of sight as much as possible.** Do not keep it on the counter or in see-through containers. Keep your healthier choices in see-through containers so you learn to choose those before the others.

9. **Do not leave bowls of small snacking foods on the counter or table.** We will eat "one or two" every time we pass.

10. **Use these principles at work, too.** Take all snacks out of your drawers and off of your desk, including candy dishes for "clients or coworkers."

11. **Bring healthy snacks and meals with you to work so you will not be at the mercy of the cafeteria, fast food, or vending machines.**

12. **Do not eat lunch at your desk.** Go to the lunchroom or a picnic table outside, but break the psychological connection between your desk and eating.

13. **At break time, avoid the break room where others may be eating or where vending machines are located.** Instead, take a stroll outside or inside your building. Make phone calls, do some stretching, exercise, or balance your checkbook.

14. **Learn to change your routine.** If you go to the refrigerator first thing after work, learn to go directly to another room so you will eventually break that connection.

15. **Learn to read labels on grocery store items.** Shop only when you are not hungry, and bring a prepared list. Avoid certain aisles that might be tempting for you, like the crackers and cookies aisle, for example. There will be little or no food appropriate for a new bariatric patient in that aisle.

16. **Play soothing music while eating.** It tends to slow us down.

17. **Try not to nibble while preparing foods.** This is a common trap. We may not eat much at dinner, but we do not count all those bites taken during preparation. Plan ahead so you are not hungry while preparing meals, and try brushing your teeth or keeping sugar-free hard candy around if you need something.

18. **If munching while you cook is a problem for you, try to prepare several meals at once to decrease the amount of time you will be vulnerable.**

19. **Keep healthy snacking alternatives available, such as sugar-free hard candies, sugar-free popsicles, or sugar-free flavored gelatin.**

20. **Always keep a bottle of water with you.** It will keep you feeling fuller between meals and is very healthy.

21. **Always have an escape route.** Do not put yourself in a situation where you feel unable to control your eating. If you find yourself

overwhelmed at any time, have a plan for how you will allow yourself to leave.

22. **Monitor your progress.** Assess your body mass index (BMI) on a monthly basis or every six months. Weigh yourself weekly or even daily. Keep track of your workouts. Many people have difficulty when they stop monitoring themselves. We tend to feel more responsible for eating and exercise when we have to be held accountable. Monitor your workouts and weight forever.

23. **Be aware of visual cues for eating.** Let's say someone puts doughnuts on a desk nearby you at work or there is a community candy bowl you pass by several times a day. A little snack here and there may feel like nothing, but it all adds up. Break the connection between eating and the cue. Move the doughnuts to another part of the office. Get rid of the candy dish. If you find your cue is being with a particular friend, then attempt to alter the connection by going to a movie instead of dinner.

24. **When you have a craving, try waiting for 10 minutes before you eat anything.** When you do not immediately respond to cravings, they tend to decrease in intensity. If you do this over time, the craved food will lose its strength and power over you.

BEHAVIOR MODIFICATION ROADBLOCKS

Behavior modification is a challenge we all must conquer to succeed in changing our old habits. Place roadblocks in your way to help you quit negative automatic behaviors, and take roadblocks out of your way to help clear the way for new positive behaviors until they can become your automatic behaviors.

Knowing it is human nature to skip workouts and stop watching our diets, proper application of the roadblocks concept can help. Figure out what obstacles keep you from success, and remove these obstacles. Also figure out the automatic habits that have lead you to skip workouts and dieting.

Examples:

1. **"I can't exercise because I don't have time to go to the gym."** Solution: remove the roadblock of limiting yourself to the gym. Instead of an expensive gym membership, buy a treadmill or an exercise bicycle for your home. You've eliminated the roadblock of driving to the gym or being limited by the gym's hours of operation.

2. **"I always overeat because it tastes so good, and I don't want the food to go to waste."** Solution: make a plate with the proper amount of food, wrap up any extra and put it in the freezer before you sit down. To have more, you must go through several steps, and at any one of those steps you can ask yourself, "Do I really want to do this?" This technique gives you a chance to decrease impulse eating by putting roadblocks in your path. Even better, take a stroll after dinner. Then clean up the kitchen after your walk when you've had a chance to relax and feel full. You can make less food to begin with if you know leftovers call your name.

Case Study

Stuart always had a bowl of ice cream after dinner. His usual routine was to move to the living room, turn on the television, and at the first commercial go to the kitchen for ice cream. When he tried to stop having ice cream after dinner in the past, he would go to the living room, watch TV, and at the first commercial he would feel extreme anxiety and anger and usually have the ice cream anyway to rid himself of these feelings. He began to think the ice cream was in charge. In just about every other diet he tried over the years, it was always the ice cream that turned out to be the problem. First he would have just a few bites per evening, then a small bowl, eventually his usual serving, and that of course led to quitting the diet altogether.

Stuart came to my office for help. He wanted to change, but it was just too difficult. He desperately wanted it to work this time, so before the surgery he was determined to control the problem. The environmental triggers were just too overwhelming for him. We came up with a plan to solve this problem.

First, he would not sit down to watch television after eating and instead would take the dog for a stroll after dinner. Second, he would make sure ice cream was not available so he could not cheat in a moment of extreme anxiety. No ice cream was allowed in his house. Third, he would learn anxiety reduction techniques, such as deep breathing and motivating self-talk, to help get him through the tough transition. Fourth, he would keep sugar-free popsicles on hand as an acceptable substitution. Fifth, he had enjoyed making model airplanes in the past and would start again so his hands would be busy while watching television.

Stuart reported a month later that it was indeed difficult, but he had been able to make the transition. This was the change he was most worried about, and when he was able to finally make it, he began to tackle other problems with similar success.

Stress Relief and Comfort Without Food

F ood is the all-American stress reliever. We eat because we are hungry, and we eat for many other recreational and emotional reasons, such as boredom, stress, excitement, tradition, habit, depression, anger, comfort, and celebration. This behavior is normal in our society, and most of us were raised this way. Just about every social activity revolves around food in some way. Food is almost always the main event. From dating, to movies, to weddings, to holidays, food is a constant. The advertising industry spends billions of dollars per year to keep all of us eating for recreational or emotional reasons.

Even though it is normal, many people have gained large amounts of weight living this way and find it very difficult to alter their lifelong habits of eating because of these emotional/recreational habits. The surgery will likely decrease your perception of hunger, but it will not help to stop your recreational or emotional eating, since this type of eating is not based on hunger cues. The key to gaining control over emotional eating is all in the mind.

Life after surgery will be stressful in ways you may not have considered. For example, what will you do on your first Thanksgiving, or your first dinner out at your favorite restaurant, or your first date? If you follow the tips provided in this book, you will most likely do well, but you will feel a heightened sense of anxiety when you cannot eat the foods you used to

...YOU WILL FEEL A HEIGHTENED sense of anxiety when you cannot eat the foods you used to love or must stop after just a couple of bites.

love, or must stop after just a couple of bites. This anxiety is normal, but you must learn some healthy ways to cope with the emotions caused by drastically altering your lifestyle.

Stress affects all of us, and some more than others. Stress is an important factor to consider when deciding whether or not to have bariatric surgery. Most people greatly underestimate the difficulty involved in drastically changing a lifestyle. How many times have you vowed to change, only to slip back into old patterns within a few months? People who are not stressed often become that way after surgery. If you are already stressed, you may become overwhelmed. How you deal with stress will either improve your ability to adhere to lifestyle changes after surgery or make it more difficult for you to achieve your goals. Stress is an eating trigger for many people. It can also make it difficult to focus on the long-term goals. Stress can make you feel tired and sap your energy and motivation, making it difficult to stick to healthy habits.

DEFAULT SETTINGS

Our comfortable old eating habits are like DEFAULT SETTINGS. When under stress, we often revert to that default setting of eating. Our default settings are the habits we try hard to resist when on a diet. They are the habits we engage in between diets. It requires focus to maintain a healthy diet and exercise routine when stressed. A crisis or big change in our lives redirects our focus, and we often begin to revert to our old habits. These default settings never really go away.

✓ TO DO

Find your own default settings by thinking about your eating patterns when you are not trying to diet. What do you eat? How much do you eat? What times of the day do you eat? These are your default habits. When you go on a diet you probably think of these, but try to resist or override them. Then, when you stop the diet, you likely return to these habits.

Example: Let's say you routinely eat pizza on Friday nights. When you go on a diet, what would you be thinking of on Friday nights? It's probably that pizza you cannot have. Once you decide you are no longer on the diet, what is the first thing you do? You probably call the pizza restaurant. It does not matter how long you stuck with the diet, there will always be a tendency to revert to your default settings.

HOW ARE OUR ORIGINAL DEFAULT SETTINGS FORMED?

Our response to food and food-related cues is established over many years and in several different ways. First, as children we may have eaten when we were upset and food calmed us down. Or we were given a bottle when we cried and then we felt better. These connections can be by chance or by design. Eventually we learned to eat in certain situations because we knew we would feel better afterward. This is a type of conditioning that strengthens over time and with repetition.

A second way we learn is by associating a food with an unrelated, separate thing, such as beer with watching football, or having doughnuts on Friday mornings at work, or having a danish while reading the newspaper. Over time, we feel compelled to do the two things together and feel anxiety if we do not.

Yet another way we learn is by listening to what our parents told us. We learned to "clean our plates," and we were being good children for doing it. We also learned by observing others. We learned that eating is a big part of celebration, family parties, a memorable Thanksgiving, and most other holidays.

These experiences form the basis of our default settings. They represent our early learning and connections that have been strengthened over many years of repetition. Breaking these connections is difficult because they are often connected to feelings of safety, security, celebration, family, and other intense emotions.

To break these habits, we must repeatedly break

the connection between the newspaper and the danish, and eventually the compulsion to eat while reading the newspaper will diminish. At the same time, a bariatric patient may begin to establish new default settings by drinking a protein shake while reading the paper.

- It is possible to set new defaults, but it takes time and conscious effort. In times of personal crisis or stress, we have a tendency to revert to the old settings. This is when it becomes important to pay special attention to our habits of eating and exercise so we will resist reverting to old habits.

DON'T EXPECT THE SURGERY to give you willpower during stressful times. It is extremely helpful to gain control over your eating before the surgery.

- Excuses are our subconscious way of allowing us to slip back to our default settings. Learn to recognize these and say NO.

In emotional situations, there can be additional stress on bariatric patients because of the conflict between wanting to eat for comfort and not wanting to cheat. Most people do not realize how stressful this is, and many people do cheat.

Don't expect the surgery to give you willpower

during stressful times. It is extremely helpful to gain control over your eating before the surgery. If you already had the surgery and are now finding yourself eating for emotional reasons, it is time to work on the problem using the techniques listed here. The surgery only keeps you from being hungry for a few months. It does nothing to stop emotional food cravings.

I ask people how they deal with stress, and almost everyone lists several healthy coping strategies. Most people also list eating as a favorite stress reducer after a hard day. Before surgery, or just after surgery, it is very important to have a few healthy coping strategies in place, or you may find yourself resorting to food for comfort. If you must eat to cope with stress, make sure it is something allowed on your diet.

HEALTHY WAYS TO DEAL WITH STRESS AND ANXIETY

Aim to utilize a few of these great stress relievers during your week.

1. Talk to a friend or family member about your feelings.
2. Spend time in a social activity not related to food.
3. Go to a movie, play, concert, or sporting event.
4. Take a leisurely drive and listen to music.
5. Go to the library, mall, or bookstore.
6. Go to the park with the dog, the kids, a friend, or alone.
7. Meditate.
8. Use Progressive Muscle Relaxation tapes (see sample script at end of chapter).

9. Exercise.
10. Do some stretching.
11. Write down your thoughts in a journal or diary.
12. Use the computer.
13. Get involved in a hobby or craft.
14. Reward yourself for all your hard work with something new.
15. Plan a vacation.
16. Get involved in a home improvement project.
17. Do some volunteer work.
18. Doodle, draw, or paint.
19. Learn a new skill, such as a sport or a language.
20. Make a list of all the things you will do when you achieve your weight goal.
21. Listen to relaxing music.
22. Use positive and motivating self-talk—give yourself a pep talk.
23. Take a hot bath.
24. Do some research on your home town and do some "tourist" activities.
25. Practice deep breathing exercises.
26. Close your eyes for a few minutes and visualize a safe, relaxing place.
27. Schedule time for yourself so you don't feel rushed.
28. Simplify your life whenever and wherever possible.

There is really no end to the possibilities. Any activity that calms you down or takes your mind off your stressors is a good choice. Whatever you do instead of eating will likely be a distant second to eating. Food has worked in the past and provided that comfort or calming effect. It may take months or even years to replace food with an acceptable alternative. A realistic expectation is that your alternative activity or relaxation technique will get your through the moment, but it will not work as well as food for some time. If you can overcome the crutch of food dependency, you will succeed.

Progressive Muscle Relaxation (PMR)

PMR is based on the fact that it is impossible to be stressed out and relaxed at the same time. Relaxation is the antidote to stress. Most of us know what it is to feel stressed and less stressed but seldom truly relaxed. PMR teaches you what complete relaxation really feels like. If you practice this several times per week for several weeks, you will be able to relax faster and will feel less stressed in situations that may cause stress for you now. Since stress is a powerful eating trigger for many people, think of PMR as a defense against emotional eating.

PMR teaches you to alternatively tense and then relax each muscle group in your body. By doing so, you will learn to relax more deeply than usual. This is helpful during the holidays, a personal crisis, or major changes in your life.

Instructions: Read the following very slowly into a tape. Pause for 3 to 5 seconds between each phrase where you see dots. Then play the tape several times per week when you can find about 12 minutes to be alone. Sit in a comfortable chair in a place relatively free of distractions.

[START OF TAPE]

Just lean back in your chair. Make yourself comfortable. Place both feet flat on the floor. Rest your hands comfortably in your lap. You may hear noises, but they will not influence your experience.

Begin by stretching your legs as far as they can go...Relax...Stretch your legs again... Point your feet up, toward you... hold...turn your feet down, away from you...hold...relax.

Now, tighten the muscles in your calves and in your thighs...tight...hold it...hold it....relax...

Feel the difference...

Let your legs go back, slowly, down to their original position...and relax all the muscles in your feet...all the muscles in your calves...and the muscles in your thighs...let your legs be completely relaxed...and now feel that wonderful relaxation coming up from your toes...up your calves...and your thighs...feeling nicely relaxed...very calm...and...very relaxed...calm and relaxed...just focus on your legs and feel your relaxation...

Now, stretch out your arms...make two fists...tighten the muscles in your fingers...feel the tightness...hold it, hold it...and relax...let your arms go down to their resting position...feel that relaxation...now stretch your arms again...tighten the muscles in your wrists, in your lower arms, in your upper arms...hold it, hold it...and, let go, just let go, let your arms go down to their original position...stop for a second, and take your time to notice that quieting feeling of relaxation through your fingers...through your hands...through your lower arms, and upper arms...let your arms go completely limp...take your time to increase that feeling of relaxation...very warm...very relaxed...calm...relaxed and calm.

Now, tighten the muscles in your back...now your chest...your abdomen...and your neck...hold it...hold it...let go of the tension. Just let go of the tension...Notice your muscles relax...take time to feel the muscles relax in your chest...in your abdomen...in your neck...all over your back...all your muscles feel nicely relaxed...

Now tighten the muscles in your face, first the muscles around your forehead, then the muscles around your eyes...make them tighter...hold it...hold it...now relax...tighten the muscles of your cheeks...the muscles around your mouth...the muscles of your chin. Make them tighter...hold it...and relax. Let all the muscles in your face relax, first the muscles of your cheeks, the muscles around your eyes, the muscles of your forehead...let all the tension drain from your face...let your chin sag if that feels good...take your time to enjoy the feeling of relaxation...very relaxed...and very calm...relaxed and calm...

Now breathe in through your nose, slowly and deeply,

and hold it...hold it...and slowly breathe out through your nose....feel the relaxation...breathe in...breathe out...relax...

Once again take a very deep breath, hold it...hold it...and slowly let it out...let go of all your tension...your frustrations...your anxieties..feeling more and more relaxed...relaxed and calm...

Now take some time to scan your body...if you notice any tense spot...take your time to release that tension...very good...very relaxed...relaxed and calm...

Now, take time to breathe in and out...slowly begin to stretch your body...when you feel ready...slowly open your eyes...and focus on your surroundings...you will be ready to continue your day...relaxed and calm..focused and attentive...[END TAPE]

Transfer of Addiction (Transfer of Vice), Alcohol, and Smoking

TRANSFER OF ADDICTION

As more and more people are undergoing bariatric surgery, previously unforeseen issues relating to the surgery are coming to light. One of these issues that is raising concern is being termed *transfer of addiction*.

Many patients have told me they traded an addiction to food for an addiction to alcohol, gambling, smoking, drugs, or shopping. Loved ones tell me, "She used to eat for stress, now she gambles." Whether a person can be "addicted" to food is still up for debate, but the word does describe how many patients feel. Transfer of addiction can be thought of as substituting addiction to eating with another undesirable behavior.

Can a person actually be addicted to food, a substance needed for survival? Research shows that some bariatric patients report experiencing addiction to food the same as a person with aloholism does with alcohol. It has not been established scientifically that a person can be "addicted" to food. The phrase comes from patients trying to describe their experiences. These patients say they feel stronger cravings than other people and have more difficulty controlling their eating. They talk about taking the substance (food) in ever increasing amounts. They try to cut down but are unable to do so for very long, and they continue to overeat in spite of the effect overeating has on health, relationships, self esteem, and work. We now know that the younger a person is when he or she becomes obese, the stronger these feelings tend to be.

Food can operate on reward centers in the brain in a way similar to drug use, which may explain the vulnerability to transfer of addiction. This may be a partly biological phenomenon, but patients also have a responsibility to protect themselves and ask for help if needed, and programs have a responsibility to educate patients.

How will a person cope with stress or emotion without food? It makes logical sense—if a person feels addicted to food and uses food in response to emotion, the addiction can change forms. I have found if a person uses food to handle stress or strong emotions, especially for a feeling of comfort, they often feel lost after surgery, searching for something to fill the void. Food may not go down, but alcohol certainly does.

HOW TO RECOGNIZE IF THERE IS A PROBLEM

1. **Take stock of your own situation.** Are you smoking? Have you started drinking alcohol? How much? Are you spending too much money? Do you feel compelled to gamble? Are you using recreational drugs?

Tip

Be extra careful if you are in recovery for drug or alcohol abuse. Right after surgery is an especially vulnerable time as you will be on pain medication in the hospital and will be sent home with a prescription. Protect yourself from falling back into those habits by and monitoring your use of medications and alcohol.

2. **Are any of these behaviors interfering with your home life, work life, relationships or health?** A drink now and then or a trip to the casino is not necessarily an issue, but once it interferes with important areas of your life it is a real problem.
3. **Has anyone close to you mentioned you may be developing a problem?**

✓ TO DO

If you think you may be headed for trouble, or perhaps have already developed an addiction, it is time to ask for help.

1. Ask the psychologist at any bariatric center for referrals and information.
2. Ask your primary care physician for referrals, medications for smoking cessation, and information.
3. Go to bariatric support groups and ask other patients how they may have handled similar problems.
4. If you need a medical detox for alcohol or drugs, call your insurance company. They can tell you the

Case Study

Gretchen weighed pounds in the second grade. At the age of 52 she had gastric bypass, lost pounds and felt great. A couple of years after surgery, she came to a group to ask for help. She had been gambling at the casino and was not winning. She said she had heard about transfer of addiction and was afraid that was what happened to her. She told the group her story. She was a comfort eater, but could not eat after surgery and she was determined to succeed. She began going with her friends to bingo as a way to occupy her time. Eventually, she upgraded to slot machines and became hooked. "At first, it was only a diversion. A hobby," she told us. Then she began going to the casino alone every weekend and sometimes during the week. When her husband threatened to leave her because of all the money she had lost, she decided to ask for help. She said it had happened so slowly that she didn't realize it was a problem until it was too late. The group brainstormed and came up with a list. First, she would plan some other activities with different people during the time she usually had free for the casino. She started out by planning dinner with relatives on the weekends. She started volunteering in the evenings so she would be occupied during the week. She gave her credit cards to her husband. She went to Gamblers Anonymous meetings twice a week. She decided to reward herself with a night at a beach hotel if she could stay away from the casino for one month. The next month she came back to announce she had been able to stick to her plan and did not go back to the casino. Every now and then Gretchen comes back to check-in. Once she even brought her husband to the group. Sometimes she does well, other times she slips. Overall she's doing much better thanks to her willingness to ask for help.

hospital they'll want you to use. Treatment will last 3 to 7 days for medical detox only, followed by some outpatient appointments. Treatment can be up to 28 days if you are interested in a longer inpatient treatment option. Call to set up an appointment to discuss it with the program administrator or counselor. If you don't have insurance, most counties have a facility that is very low cost or free. Any medical detox program can give you the number to that facility in your area.

5. If you already have a psychologist, talk to him or her about working on transfer of addiction before other issues.

6. There are resources, such as Alcoholics Anonymous (AA), Narcotics Anonymous (NA), Gamblers Anonymous, and multiple others, with convenient meetings in almost every city. There are even groups for your family members to learn how best to help you.

7. Don't put it off. These problems tend to escalate over time, so it's always better to address it sooner than later.

ALCOHOL

A survey of patients in 2006 found that after bariatric surgery patients are much more sensitive to alcohol. Most participants in the survey said they did feel increased sensitivity to alcohol. About a quarter of the participants said they had no problem with alcohol before surgery, but did develop a problem afterward. Some patients reported receiving a citation for driving while intoxicated or driving under the influence after just one drink.

Several factors may be to blame. After bypass surgery, alcohol spends less time in the stomach and

It appears that bypass patients absorb about 50 percent more alcohol for each drink consumed, and it quickly **PEAKS IN THEIR SYSTEM.**

empties quickly into the intestines where it is absorbed rapidly. In addition, bariatric patients are taught not to eat and drink at the same time, but without food in the stomach alcohol quickly empties into the intestine and is absorbed faster. It appears that bypass patients absorb about 50 percent more alcohol for each drink consumed, and it quickly peaks in their system. The result is a wallop that few people are prepared to handle.

Becoming an alcoholic is not a side effect of bariatric surgery, but there does appear to be a vulnerability for which patients should be prepared. Here's a good "rule of thumb" to go by. If you don't drink now, no need to start. If you do, two to three drinks per week after surgery is fine after goal weight is achieved, but be careful. I've heard it described by patients like this: If you like alcohol before the surgery, you will love it afterward. The danger is it's easy to become dependent on alcohol. Even people that never had a problem with alcohol can struggle with dependency after surgery.

You must be very careful with alcohol consumption after surgery. The effect is different for everybody, but for some it can be dangerous. Monitor your own habits concerning alcohol and watch out for your health and well being.

Case Study

Penny had bariatric surgery two years ago. Before surgery she had a steady boyfriend, a good job, and did not drink alcohol except on holidays. After surgery she had several complications that put her in the hospital at least twice. She had a very hard time tolerating anything other than protein shakes for months. She was a person who tended to eat for stress and bad days, but when the food was not an option she started to drink a little alcohol. It went down just fine and relaxed her as well. She began drinking more, and after six months was up to two bottles of wine per day. She ended up with ulcers and vitamin deficiencies, was admitted to the hospital, and that's where I saw her next. She told me she had lost her health, her boyfriend, and her job. While in the hospital she was motivated to change and stop drinking, but once she was discharged she started drinking again immediately. Her next admission to the hospital five months later was the final straw. She said she finally had enough, and planned to get help as soon as she was discharged. This time she followed through. Penny was able to stop drinking with the help of her doctor, her support groups, and a lot of determination to get healthy. She says it is still a struggle, but getting easier every week. She is working part-time and is back together with her boyfriend. She now knows the warning signs and says she'll never let alcohol take over her life again.

Here are some guidelines to assist you in making wise choices concerning alcohol after surgery.

1. Do not consume alcohol while losing weight. It slows down weight loss, lowers inhibition, which

leads to eating inappropriate foods, provides calories with no nutrition, and is a diuretic.

2. Once goal weight is achieved and your program's dietitian gives the go-ahead, keep it at two to three drinks per week or less, and never more than one on any day.

3. B vitamins are very important after surgery. They are even more important if you are consuming alcohol. Be careful to take all your vitamins on a daily basis.

4. Don't drink while driving, even after just one drink.

5. Eat something if you are having an alcoholic beverage.

6. If you think you may be developing a problem with alcohol, approach your program's psychologist for guidance.

SMOKING

Smoking is not uncommon before surgery. Various studies have found between 16 and 38 percent of bariatric surgery candidates are smokers. Many patients say they smoke to deal with stress or smoke to keep weight off. Some say they've quit many times in the past, only to return during very stressful times.

Most programs will want a patient to be smoke free for eight weeks before surgery. Some require up to three months, and actually test their patients before surgery. Some weight loss surgery programs will cancel a surgery if a person has started smoking again. The reason is because smokers have a higher risk for complications during surgery.

If a patient starts smoking after surgery, he or she is at higher risk for further complications and hospital readmissions.

Smoking is highly addictive. It is surprising how many patients have said, "I'm doing this surgery for my health," but they continue to smoke. Smoking is one of the worst things a person can do if health is a concern. If you are a smoker, this may be a motivation. Think about how inconsistent it is to want to have the surgery in order to improve your health and yet continue to smoke. Focus on really doing something positive for your health.

> If a patient starts smoking after surgery, he or she is at higher risk for **FURTHER COMPLICATIONS AND HOSPITAL READMISSIONS.**

Smoking can be so addictive that some people will smoke when it is incredibly detrimental to their health, and even ignore multiple doctors' orders. If you are one of those people, get some professional assistance in quitting.

Quitting is very hard to do, and quit rates are low. They are significantly higher with new medications. If you are a smoker, discuss with your doctor the possibility of a trial on one of those new medications.

Internal motivation to quit appears to be the factor most responsible for successful quitting. Interestingly, people that just decide they have had enough and decide to quit have higher success rates. Many people have said they just quit "cold turkey."

Quitting is only half of the challenge. Staying abstinent is tough. People are at a high risk for relapse when they feel they have successfully stopped smoking. "I can handle it now, I'll just have one cigarette." Stress is another red flag. We tend to justify cigarettes "because it's just so stressful right now." Once you stop, maintenance becomes very important.

How to Quit:

1. Talk to your doctor about assistance in the form of information, medication, and/or nicotine-replacement recommendations.
2. Consider joining a smoking cessation program. A list will be available from your insurance provider.
3. Seek assistance on the Internet. Good websites include the following:
   a. www.smokefree.gov
   b. www.cdc.gov/tobacco/
   c. www.lungusa.org
   d. www.americanheart.org
4. Get your family involved. Ask that others not smoke around you.
5. Think about your health.
6. Change your habits. If you smoke after dinner, then have a piece of sugar-free hard candy after dinner or brush your teeth right away. If you smoke in the car, minimize time in the car, sing instead of smoke, and clean your car so that it smells fresh.
7. You will experience anxiety. It cannot hurt you.
8. Once you have gone three days, you are a nonsmoker.

Weight Maintenance

Weight loss attempts are complicated by many factors. The media entice us with mouth-watering commercials and ads depicting young, fit, happy people having fun and eating double bacon cheeseburgers. These images make us want to eat. Food is the main event in most social events ranging from baseball games, to weddings, to dating. Our environment makes it very difficult to maintain weight loss after we achieve our weight goal and begin to eat more again.

When we are not eating or thinking about eating, we are often dieting, reading about dieting, or planning our next one. The diet business is thriving. There are hundreds of diets available, and most will help you lose weight. Very few will help you understand the value of weight maintenance. We all seem very good at being on diets and just as good at being off diets, but not very good at maintenance.

People lose weight all the time, but usually gain it back as soon as they stop the diet. How many times have you lost weight vowing to never gain it back, then one day you notice it's back? No one ever goes into bariatric surgery planning to regain weight either. Before surgery, just about everyone says, "If I can just get the weight off, I'll do everything in my power to keep it off." Yet, weight regain does happen. It is poor post-diet maintenance that causes people to gain the weight back. For those of you considering weight loss surgery, maintenance has to be your ultimate goal. You will lose weight if you follow the diet after surgery, but maintenance is a lifelong challenge even for bariatric patients. Many people do gain some or all the weight back after surgery, so learning the proper steps in weight maintenance is very important.

There is an incredibly strong pull to go back to our old eating habits. They are comfortable and familiar, and they just feel right. The habits are forged over

PEOPLE LOSE WEIGHT ALL THE TIME

but usually gain it back...It is poor post-diet maintenance that causes people to gain the weight back. For those of you considering weight loss surgery, maintenance has to be your ultimate goal.

many years. Think of your old eating habits as your default settings. You will want to revert to those default settings when under stress or when you reach your weight loss goal. Weight maintenance means resisting those urges to slip back into old eating patterns. It is an ongoing process that may be difficult in the beginning, but as you learn and practice these techniques, they will become second nature to you. Over many months and years, you can adjust your default settings. Just because you may have gained the weight back before does not mean that you will again.

PSYCHOLOGICAL BASICS OF WEIGHT MAINTENANCE IN THAT "IN-BETWEEN" STATE

So you've lost the weight. Congratulations! You have been through some very difficult situations and have been successful. Now your focus has to shift to weight maintenance.

We have been conditioned to be either "on" or "off" a diet. This is called "all-or-nothing" thinking. This type of thinking usually leads to yo-yo dieting as we continually go on and off diets, losing, gaining, and then losing weight again and again. We are comfortable trying to diet, and comfortable not dieting, but somewhat uneasy in that in-between state of maintenance. It is called the "in-between" state because you may eat a bit more, but must not revert to old eating habits. Your challenge is to develop a whole new mindset. It will become your new default setting. With this mindset, you will always be on a diet to some extent because you will always be watching your food intake.

With maintenance, the diet is less strict. You have some leeway in what you eat and can eat a few more calories, but do not think of yourself as being "off" the diet. It is helpful to think of a weight problem as a chronic health issue that you will have for the rest of your life. With your procedure (your assistant) you can control it, but the weight can always come back. The surgery doesn't change your genes, the environment, your own cravings, your urges, your emotional eating, or your early learning. If you forget where you came from, you may be at risk to regain. Try to look at the following four things daily, and you'll have an excellent chance to keep the weight down and live a healthy life:

1. Watch your food intake. Be self-sufficient, plan ahead, have your food with you.

2. Continue your exercise program—for life. Keep an exercise log and exercise daily or close to it for life.

3. Weigh yourself weekly or even daily for the rest of your life.

4. Keep your environment set up for success. Remember—we all eat "whatever's there," so make sure that "whatever" is bariatric friendly. Minimize trigger foods in your home.

Your program's dietitian and surgeon will provide information on your maintenance diet food choices. Watch out for the tendency to overeat. This is a time when some people really let down their guard, so be careful. Our tendency is to reach the goal and then go "off" the diet. How you handle this time is critical for long-term success.

The point at which you are reaching your weight goal is a dangerous time. This is when it is natural to start to feel like "everyone else." You see everyone else can eat fast food and skip the exercise. You will appear like everyone else on the outside, but you are not. Don't ever lose sight of that fact, or you will be in danger of slipping back into your old habits.

You should be exercising at least three times per week. I recommend five times or more if possible. Once you reach your goal weight and maintenance begins, you may feel the urge to stop exercising. This will put you at risk to gain weight back. Exercise

> **YOU WILL APPEAR LIKE EVERYONE ELSE** on the outside, but you are not. Don't ever lose sight of that fact, or you will be in danger of slipping back into your old habits.

must continue indefinitely in order to keep the weight off. It is a very important component to weight maintenance. If you experience a drop in motivation to continue exercising, be sure to reread the motivational section of this book and talk to a friend. If all else fails, please make an appointment with a psychologist.

When you get to the weight maintenance stage, you must also continue to watch your food intake. This book does not go into detail on the science of weight maintenance, but rather discusses the psychological techniques to help keep you on track. Most bariatric surgery candidates have not had success at maintenance and have usually lost and gained weight many times. You may think the most difficult part of weight loss was the surgery, but weight maintenance has its own set of challenges.

Psychologically, you feel like you have completed your task. The weight is off, you are feeling better, you are looking better, and you have a better mental outlook. Expect your self-talk to go something like this: "I can afford to take a couple of weeks off from exercising now, just a short vacation. I deserve it. I'll start again in 10 days." Beware. You have just taken the first step to a complete exercise meltdown. Chances are slim that you will soon start again. Do not fall into this trap. It is difficult to really motivate yourself to start an exercise program, so don't ever let it stop. If you experience a stressful period in your life, just cut back to two workouts per week. When the crisis passes, go back to your usual three to five times per week.

✓ TO DO

1. **Come to terms with the fact that if you want to keep the weight off, exercise must become a permanent part of your life.** Like brushing your teeth or taking a shower, it is an essential activity that is here to stay. Many psychologists believe we are "hard-wired" to say YES to food and NO to exercise.

2. **Do not believe the excuses and self-talk you tell yourself in order to avoid exercise.** Taking time off is a red flag. Your task is to motivate yourself. Remember how far you have come, and don't let anything stand in the way of your exercise.

3. **For some, it is easier to be "on" or "off" a diet than being on a maintenance diet because you have more choices.** Get yourself under control if you notice that you are cheating too much. Relocate your "middle ground."

4. **Realize you will never eat like others again.** You are different and have special needs and considerations. Make peace with this, and you will feel less anxiety over your differences. Try to look at your uniqueness as a positive. After all, look where it got you.

5. **Keep your eye on the scale.** Weigh yourself at least weekly. If you notice a few pounds of weight gain, it may just be the time of day or expected fluctuations in weight. If you notice a trend over a couple of weeks, take action. Sit down and plan your meals and exercise and get back on track. Getting back to basics is usually a good place to start. This means checking your environment for trigger foods and keeping your exercise consistent. Begin using your food and exercise log books again.

6. **Positive self-talk will be important for the rest of your life.** Tell yourself you are worth the time and that you will not backslide.

7. **Try to be self sufficient with your food because it is not a bariatric friendly world.**

8. **You may have to avoid some foods forever because of the hold they have over you.** The goal is to protect yourself from certain foods or

situations when you know it might be difficult to control eating. Other patients find they are able to eat anything in moderation. If this does not work for you, perhaps you just traded a few foods for better health, mobility, and quality of life.

9. **As always, if you are unable to gain control or motivate yourself, please call a psychologist for help.** After thousands of dollars in medical care and countless days and hours working toward your goal, do not jeopardize what you have accomplished. Call for help if you need it. Often, it is just a few weeks of assistance and you will be back on top.

Tips on Long-term Maintenance and Revisions

According to many patients, it's easier to adhere to lifestyle changes while losing weight and in the first couple of years after achieving goal weight than during the long-term maintenance phase. During active weight loss, patients feel excited and amazed at the things they can do. They buy new wardrobes, start relationships, and get lots of positive feedback from friends, family, and coworkers. This is the time when weight loss and weight maintenance is foremost on the mind.

Fast-forward 10, 20, 30 years or more and a different picture emerges. The pouch may have expanded, allowing larger meals. The negative physical feedback a person gets when he or she eats too fast, too much, or the wrong foods may be nonexistent or greatly diminished. Dumping syndrome may be gone as well. The "little policeman" as one of my patients describes it, has retired. Perhaps you can't even remember being heavy because you had surgery so many years ago. No one comments on the weight anymore. The fashionable clothes you bought years ago are now outdated, and it's no longer exciting. It's just normal life.

The maintenance phase can be 50 years or more. During this time, the focus needs to change. In order to remain successful, a person's lifestyle changes must

Weight maintenance is not the only

MEASURE OF SUCCESS.

continue indefinitely. The natural human tendency is to slack off. You may feel like changes you made can continue on autopilot. How do you increase the likelihood of keeping most of the weight off? The answer is to continue lifestyle changes indefinitely and proactively monitor your health.

Weight maintenance is not the only measure of success. Most people will gain back 20 to 40 pounds, which is normal over time. Other measures of success are decreased disability and disease, increased mobility, and increased quality of life on many levels. A person may find he or she can walk again, go back to work, play with the kids, and tie his or her own shoes. Even with some regain, a person may still experience these positive effects of weight loss. There is no reason to panic if you experience a normal amount of weight gain over the years. There are things you can do to assist in maintaining your higher quality of life. Don't obsess about a few pounds weight gain if you believe your quality of life remains good.

Case Study

Christopher was a very successful bariatric patient. When I met him he had lost 160 pounds and maintained it for 10 years. Christopher did everything right. He always took food with him wherever he went so he would not have to find bariatric appropriate food when he got hungry. This simple technique helped him stay in charge and on track. One day he came to the group in a panic. He had regained 20 pounds. He said his family told him he didn't need to bring his food with him any longer. He needed to move on, and to get over the surgery. He listened to them, and began leaving his cooler at home. Over the next few months he started eating foods he had been avoiding, and started putting on weight. In the group we suggested he go back to bringing his food with him. At first he had a hard time with that suggestion as he thought it might alienate his family. By the time the group was over he had committed to taking back his health by using the techniques that made him successful in the first place. He took the weight off in no time by deciding to take back control.

Other people may not understand what a bariatric patient has to go through, so trust yourself and your own habits. If it works for you, keep doing it.

✓ TO DO

1. **Self-monitor—forever.** Research shows consistently that people who make themselves accountable by monitoring themselves do better, lose more, and maintain weight loss longer. Slipping back into old habits usually happens slowly, a little here, a little there, a bite here, and a pound there. If you're not paying attention it can sneak up on you.

2. Keep logs.

A. Keep an exercise log for life. Use it as an early warning system. It will tell you if exercise is slipping. Try to exercise five times per week or more for life.

B. Keep a weight log and check your weight on a weekly or daily basis. This will also act as an early warning system and will signal if there is a problem developing.

3. Go to support groups on a regular basis. It is not necessary to go constantly, but at least a couple times per year. It's good to remind yourself what you've been through, where you came from, and how you are different. Go back to support groups if you've gotten away or if one of your early warning systems highlights a problem (stopped exercising or gained a significant amount of weight).

4. Pick a date during the year to use as a prompt, perhaps the anniversary of your surgery. Use this target date to get your annual blood work done, to get your vitamin levels checked, and to go to an anniversary support group. Recommit to a healthy lifestyle.

5. Use the target date to evaluate your adherence to your program.

A. Are you exercising enough?

B. Are you following the maintenance diet? Have you started to go back to old habits?

C. Is your environment still set up to help you? Or have some of those old favorite foods come back into the house?

D. Formulate a plan for the next year, addressing any problems you identify.

Case Study

Barbara had slowly regained 35 pounds after losing 180 pounds 10 years ago. Although this is normal, she wanted to take most of it back off. Her goal to "just lose the weight" was not helping to motivate her. When she looked below the surface about why she wanted to lose the weight, her motivation became clear. She wanted to feel more comfortable on her beach vacation and maybe even try parasailing. With this motivating thought, she was able to succeed in her weight loss. She went to Cancun with her family and did try parasailing. When she returned she began looking for new goals to keep her motivated.

E. Think of it like a spring-cleaning. Take stock of your situation and make any adjustments necessary to get yourself back on track.

6. **Stay connected to the bariatric community.** Visit websites, chat online, keep up with new research, subscribe to magazines, read new books, and check out new products. The bariatric field is growing rapidly, and new products and magazines are hitting the shelves on a regular basis.

7. **Address any relapse as soon as possible.**

8. **Don't lie to yourself that you don't have to worry about weight anymore.** You will always have a weight problem, but you can control it with your behaviors and your procedure. If you let down your guard, and decide you no longer have to worry about it, you are at risk of gaining the weight back, and losing your higher quality of life.

Case Study

Diane had gastric bypass in 1985. Her weight went from 360 to 170, but she slowly regained over the years. She needed to take off 90 pounds to get back to her most comfortable weight of 170 pounds. Back in 1985, there were no large bariatric centers, and the education given to patients was much different than it is now. Diane said, "They just gave me the surgery and told me to take my vitamins. No one even mentioned exercise or what to eat for the rest of my life." She said she was trying to lose weight on her own, but found out her pouch was now enlarged and she needed a revision. She did have the revision and has been able to lose 60 pounds so far. She is happy with the results, and her high blood pressure has retreated as well. This time she has all the information she needs to be successful in the long run, and she is committed to making it work.

9. **Use self-talk to motivate yourself.** Say things like "I may not like to exercise, but it sure is nice to be able to do it. I'm never going back." Motivation for weight loss has probably been nonexistent for many years, so you must do whatever it takes to get jumpstarted again.

10. **Do what works.** Only you know what works for you. Your "Success Habits" are yours alone. What works for you may not work for the next guy. It doesn't matter if you are watching your diet for three months or for the rest of your life. Similarly, when you stop with your success habits, you will stop being successful. Maybe what helps you to be successful is shopping with a list, keeping certain foods out of the house, avoiding certain restaurants, exercising at a specific time, and taking your lunch to work.

Marcy's Letter

Marcy is a post-op patient. She had surgery over six years ago and has kept all of her weight off. Marcy is a regular in my Emotional Wellness Groups at Cleveland Clinic, and she always has great advice. She came up with a system to help her stay at her goal weight, and it was so creative I asked her if it could be included in the book. The following is her advice for long-term weight maintenance in her own words:

"I started with the question 'How am I going to maintain at my goal weight?' I knew that I could lose weight because I had lost over 100 pounds several times in my life; unfortunately, I was never able to keep it off for very long. I was so sure there was an easy answer out there somewhere. But now that it's been nearly six years since my weight loss surgery, with nearly four and a half years at my goal weight, I've come to the conclusion that the answer for me is sticking to the BASICS:

B is for BREATHE. Having a history of eating to relieve anxiety, I need to take deep breaths when I feel stressed and wait for the urge to eat to pass. I can do it anywhere, anytime, with no equipment needed.

A is for ACTIVITY. I know I feel better when I do at least 30 minutes of cardio every day. It curbs my appetite and lowers my stress level. My goal is to exercise 5 to 7 days a week.

S is for supplements. I hate pills so I take supplements in liquid form whenever possible; it's so easy to forget to take them, but not when I use my checkoff list.

I is for I (ME). I need to do these basic things before I attempt to save the rest of the world; whatever I put in front of my basic needs, I'll lose anyway. I function best in a clean, orderly environment—be it my house, my car, my papers.

C is for CALORIES and CARBS. I know I need to keep my daily calories below 1900; that is easier to do when I limit my carbs to less than 100g a day (keeps the cravings down). I do better when I have mostly protein and salad during the day and limit my starchy carbs and fruit to the evening. I have a major memory block on how much I eat, so I HAVE to write it down. I haven't had sugar or flour since my surgery and my fear of where it could take me leaves me "scared straight."

S is for SLEEP. I do best with eight hours of sleep a night. I also do better when I go to bed at 10:30 and get up at 6:30. My worst eating bouts take place after 10:30 p.m.

The bottom line? The good news is that I finally have an answer on how to stay thin. The bad news is that its not easy. And it's not like I just have to struggle with the decision once—I have to redecide every day, all day long. It could be overwhelming except that all I need to do is make the right choice 18 out of 20 times, which is 90 percent of the time—still an A!

11. **Don't listen to anyone who tells you to stop worrying about your weight or tries to change you or your habits**. You know better.

12. **If your motivation to continue is diminished, set new goals.** Challenge yourself by learning a new sport or rewarding yourself with something really special like a trip. Keep moving the finish line. Motivation must be manufactured every day; it doesn't happen automatically.

13. **Look beyond the weight.** Focus on the quality of your life and how you feel.

14. **Be protective of your own success habits.** They will serve you forever.

15. Use technology to your advantage. Set up reminders on your mobile device that delivers prompts for shopping, vitamins, exercise, support groups, and doctors appointments. Set up an annual prompt for blood work and doctor appointment.

REVISIONS

It's possible to have a surgical revision. This can sometimes be done in response to weight regain or if a person does not lose enough weight after the first procedure.

The overall goal is to avoid having to have a revision if possible. In general, risks are higher with revisions than with the original procedure. A higher percentage of surgeries must be done open instead of laproscopically, and there is a higher incidence of leaks and infection. Because of this it is advisable to consider a revision only as a last resort.

Additional Tips for Success

AVOIDING THE RED ZONE (Logic vs. Emotion)

Many people think that when it comes to food, they can just "make better choices." Sounds great but it's not that simple. Where we are when we make those choices, how hungry we are, and what our emotions are at the time all impact our ability to make good decisions. Making a better or different choice is easier if we are far away from food, or if we are not extremely hungry. The objective, well-reasoned choice can only take place under those circumstances. Once we're in front of food or very hungry, we are no longer making objective choices, but purely emotional choices. This is called the "red zone," the danger area, where objectivity concerning food goes out the window. We are much more likely to eat something then regret it while in the red zone. An example may be your favorite restaurant, a wedding reception, or a family holiday party.

The following tips can help you avoid the red zone and make better choices:

1. Think in terms of self-protection. Try to avoid putting yourself in the red zone by planning ahead and not allowing yourself to become famished.

2. Before you go to a restaurant, check the menu online. See if there's something you can order, and make up your mind before you go. Once in the restaurant, the sights and smells will take over and possibly sway your resolve, so have a plan already in place when you arrive.

3. The worst thing to do is show up unprepared, try to wing it, and say to yourself, "I'll just make better choices." The red zone is very powerful.

FAST FOOD

Fast food tends to be a staple in many patients' diets prior to surgery. It's understandable as fast food is convenient, filling, tasty, inexpensive, and you don't even have to get out of your car. Unfortunately, there are few fast foods that are really acceptable for a bariatric patient.

Fast food is one area that really gets people in trouble after surgery. Often weight regain is a direct result of patients going back to fast-food rationalizing: "I don't have time for anything else."

SECRET OF SUCCESSFUL PATIENTS

There is one thing faster than fast food, and that is having all your food with you. Be self sufficient. A successful bariatric patient is visible from a great distance, not because of how he or she looks, but because he or she will have a rolling suitcase or a cooler with him or her wherever the patient goes. He or she will always have cheese sticks, yogurt, protein bars, and water with him or her. That way he or she will not have to rely on chance or luck for his or her food choices. The successful bariatric patient will not have to worry about what restaurant he or she will pass on the way home, because he or she has complete control.

TIPS ON HOW TO BE SUCCESSFUL

1. We will lie to ourselves to go to a fast food restaurant, and say something like, "I'll just get a salad." But when the server asks if you want fries with that, you're in trouble. That's because you are in the red zone. It's next to impossible to make a healthy choice in this situation. We may go there with the best intentions, but it's hard to choose the salad when your favorite sandwich and fries are on the menu. It's a good idea to make a rule that if you find yourself out and about without your own food, you'll go to a grocery store and get quarter pound of sliced turkey at the deli. Don't leave the possibility open for fast food.

2. Some of us actually set ourselves up by getting up late, saying "Oh well, now I <u>have</u> to get fast food." The incentives to "forget" to plan ahead are stacked in the favor of fast food. Change the incentives so if you forget to prepare, you must go to the deli at the grocery store, not the fast food restaurant. If you are one of those people who is always late for work and simply can't get up early to pack a lunch, then do it

the night before when you have time. Preload your life. Then all you have to do is grab the cooler and you're ready to go.

3. The fast food industry hires psychologists to help convince you to eat their food. The owners of these restaurants get stock options and new yachts when they are successful; you get extra pounds and declining health. It doesn't seem like a fair tradeoff. Say to yourself, "I'm not going to help them get rich at the expense of my health any longer." Fight back against the millions of dollars spent each year to convince us that fast food is great.

4. Many people who eat fast food on a regular basis have a difficult time keeping their weight in the normal range, and health problems often follow the weight gain. Although fast food every now and then is not the end of the world, it can lead to weight regain if it becomes a dietary staple. There are millions of people who <u>never</u> eat at fast food restaurants.

5. With fast food, we don't pay with time or money—we pay with poor health and weight gain. Decide ahead of time which way you would like to pay.

SKILLS TRANSFER

It would be impossible to count the number of patients who have said, "I've been successful in every other area of my life, but I just can't stick with a diet or exercise program." When asked what gets in the way, they say "I guess I'm just lazy," or "I don't have willpower." It doesn't matter if you're a CEO, doctor, lawyer, business owner, or other highly accomplished

Case Study

Jack had a habit before surgery of always stopping at the donut shop for coffee and a couple of donuts on the way to work. After surgery he stopped doing that, lost weight to his goal and kept it off for 2 years. He said he "never felt better." His life changed as he ended up getting a new job, and was in a new relationship. Something changed about 3 years after surgery. He started to gain weight. He said he had gone back to his coffee at the donut shop, but that wasn't the problem. While he was waiting in the drive-thru, his resolve disappeared, and he started ordering donuts. Once he started, he said he just couldn't stop. He would put himself in the donut shop drive-thru every morning, determined to just order coffee, then he ended up ordering donuts, eating them, and feeling guilty for the rest of the day. His family tried to help him stop by talking to him on the phone on the way to work. Eventually he just turned the phone off to go to the drive-thru. He gained over 50 lbs. before he got scared and came back to groups. He was able to make changes by making a rule that he would not go, by making coffee at home and taking it to work, by having breakfast before he left the house so he was not hungry, and taking a different route to work. He wasn't perfect as he did slip five times during that first month, but he kept coming back to groups and kept picking himself up after every slip and making changes. He lost about half of the weight he gained, and still struggles with the donuts. He told me recently that he does still stop there about twice per month, but at least now it isn't every day.

person. If you have achieved a high level of success with work, school, or family, you are anything but lazy. If this sounds like you, the following section may help to transfer that success to this project.

Highly successful people have one thing in common. They succeed because they have certain traits, skills, and strengths that they apply to work, home, school, and/or family. Success has followed because they use these strengths to their advantage. They are guilty of having a double standard, however, which is having one set of rules for work, school, or family, and another set for diet and exercise. Here's how:

To be a successful CEO for example, a person must be organized, set priorities, persist in the face of adversity, and stick with it day after day regardless of mood or energy level. How successful would that CEO be if he had used the same standard he might use for exercise? For example, if he said at work, "I'm not motivated to go to that meeting today," or, "I worked really hard yesterday so I'm just going to rest today," or "I really don't want to do that paperwork today. I'm just not in the mood." Approaching your diet and exercise in the same light as you approach your other life successes is not a far reach. Apply the strengths that got you where you are in work, school, or family, to this particular project. Thinking of lifestyle changes, such as diet and exercise adherence, as a second job is a comfortable place for many high achieving people as they already have the tools to be successful.

✓ TO DO

1. Make a list of those qualities, skills, strengths, and traits that make you successful in other areas of your life. How can you use these to assist you with diet and exercise?

2. Hold yourself accountable. Monitor your progress, exercise, and weight on paper.

3. Prioritize behaviors that lead to success; don't make exercise optional.

4. Approach diet and exercise as a second job. Don't rely on chance, mood, energy level, or motivation to engage in the actions that will make you successful in this endeavor.

CHAINING

Chaining is an interesting psychological phenomenon that occurs naturally in our daily lives. Chaining happens when several behaviors become linked over time, making it natural to do them together the same way. Using this technique, pathways can actually be created in the brain making it easier to stick to your bariatric routines. Consider applying chaining to post-operative, self-care behaviors to help you with long-term habit change. Here are some examples of chaining:

1. You get in your car, close the door, put on the seatbelt, put the key in the ignition, press the gas pedal, and turn the key. You don't have to think about any of these steps because you've done it the same way thousands of times. All you have to do is just get in the car, and it triggers the other behaviors.

2. You dial a phone number so many times, you may not remember the number, but if you go to dial it, your fingers remember.

3. You turn on the water and get into the shower. You don't have to think about what you will wash next as your hands have done it thousands of times. You

can think about vacation, and you will automatically finish showering without missing anything.

This concept can be applied to diet and exercise to help you establish your new habits.

✓ TO DO

Come up with a routine you can live with. For example, you get up, exercise, take a shower, have a protein shake, take your vitamins, sit down to read the paper. If you spend the next six months doing this every day the same way, eventually just getting up will trigger the rest of the chain, making it easier to stick with your plan. There are so many details to worry about as a bariatric patient, and developing a predictable chain of behaviors will help.

STRUCTURE

Structure makes it easier to stick with habits. People who have retired or are not working have more flexibility in their schedules. Although this can be a good thing, it can also lead to putting things off. Retirees can sleep late, worry about cutting the grass tomorrow, and enjoy the day. This is a double-edged sword because this lack of structure can lead to difficulty sustaining lifestyle changes.

Human beings are creatures of habit. We like routines. When we have too much flexibility in our schedule, sometimes we have the tendency to put things off. If you are one of the lucky ones that has retired, try to place structure in your life and adhere to a set of rules to assist with all the changes you are making. Try to get up at the same time and work out early in the day. Shop and plan meals on a regular basis, and take your vitamins at specific times during the day. If you stick with it, your routine will become second nature over time.

Some retirees find themselves staying up later and later, and perhaps napping during the day. If this applies to you, it will be helpful to put yourself on a more predictable sleep/wake cycle.

✓ TO DO

Start getting up at the same time every day, preferably early in the morning. Don't worry about what time you go to sleep this first week. Try to avoid napping during the day. Within a week or so, you will find yourself falling asleep at an earlier hour, and this will normalize your sleep pattern.

Case Study

Jake spent most of his life in the military. When he retired he looked forward to having time on his hands. He was able to keep his weight under control in the military, which he credited to the structure and routine of military life. When he retired, he gained 140 pounds in just over five years. Jake enjoyed his postmilitary life, and all the freedom and flexibility that came with it. All this free time contributed to his weight gain because he never seemed to get around to exercise and had time to eat out more often. Jake understood that to be successful after weight loss surgery, he would need to get back to some of the routines he had in the military. He started getting up at the same time every day and doing his exercise before anything else. He ate three meals a day and always at the same time. He chose two days per week when he would plan his upcoming meals and go to the market. He took care of all his bariatric-related tasks before noon, then allowed himself to have fun in the afternoon. Jake said the structure he created felt right, and having routines made it easier for him. Jake is doing well these days. He has taken off over 100 pounds and credits adding structure to his life as a major component in his success.

Relapse Prevention

elapse prevention is a term used by psychologists to describe a new perspective for a common reaction. Think of how many times you may have been watching your diet, had a bad day, ate something you regretted, and then said, "Well, I have blown it now. I might as well have some ice cream, too." Human beings have a tendency to try to be perfect, and if we aren't, then we just go back to our old habits. We call this "all-or-nothing thinking." It just means we either watch our diets perfectly or we don't watch at all. An important key to long-term weight maintenance is learning relapse prevention techniques. These allow you to stay on your diet even though you may have eaten something you regret. They teach you to ignore "all-or-nothing" thinking.

✓ TO DO

1. **Realize no one is perfect.** You are not a robot. Do not expect to be 100-percent adherent to your bariatric diet.

2. **When you do "slip," you then have a choice.** You can either revert to the old eating patterns of the past and eventually begin to gain weight or learn from the "slip." Ask yourself some questions: Why did it happen? What can I learn from it so I will not make this mistake in the future?

3. **Stop the thoughts that say, "I already blew it. I'll start again Monday."** If you forget to brush your teeth on Wednesday, would you wait until Monday to start again? Replace that thinking with, "I only ate one piece of candy. It was 600 calories. I will not let this ruin all my progress. I am in charge." Use positive self-talk to your advantage. It is easier to stop yourself after one or two slips than after letting go for weeks or months.

4. **Recognize that there is no end to a lifestyle change. It will go on forever.**

5. **Focus on the big picture.** In any lifestyle change, there is a general trend toward success, but there are hundreds of daily and weekly ups and downs. Do not focus on the tiny ups and downs, but rather the big picture.

6. **Try to get an "A minus" in lifestyle change.** If you strive for perfection, you set yourself up for

failure as this is not possible. Instead, strive for an A minus. This means that 9 times out of 10 you follow the rules, but every now and then it's OK to slip.

7. **The old thinking may have been, "If I fall off the wagon I've blown it. I might as well forget it and eat what I want. This won't work."** A healthier approach is much more realistic. You will fall off the wagon thousands of times between now and the end of your life. Falling off the wagon is not the problem. It never has been. It's how long you stay off that's the problem. If you can get back on track the next meal or the next day, you'll be fine. If you wait six months, you won't be fine, and you will gain a lot of weight during that time. It's not the piece of birthday cake that's the problem, it's the downward slide afterward because you've "blown it."

Try a new mindset. Take your thinking from "If this doesn't work, I'll just go back to my old habits," to "No matter what happens I will get back on the horse. I will be successful and not let small slips keep me from my goal of lifelong good health and excellent quality of life." Lifestyle changes never end.

EMERGENCY FIRST AID KIT

There will be times when you completely fall off the wagon. You slip into your old, comfortable eating pattern and stop exercising. This is when a slip or a lapse becomes a full-fledged relapse. Perhaps it will be a family crisis, relocation, or major change in your job. When this happens, it is time to go BACK TO BASICS.

Basics of Your Emergency First Aid Kit:

1. Scrutinize your environment for obstacles and take all trigger foods out of the house. We tend to eat "whatever's there," so make sure "whatever's there" are healthy choices.

2. Commit to monitoring yourself until you feel confident:
   a. Weigh yourself weekly.
   b. Start a new daily food log.
   c. Start a new daily exercise log.

3. Exercise immediately to reestablish the habit.

4. Set up rewards for exercise.

5. Shop for healthy foods and snacks.

6. Use positive self-talk. Remember where you started.

7. Look at your habits, roadblocks, and obstacles to success. Rearrange and prioritize.

8. Contact a local bariatric program for support groups and attend several meetings.

Almost everyone will experience these episodes. Your choice is always to continue down that path or to use your Emergency First Aid Kit.

Relationships and How They May Change After Surgery

Most bariatric patients never consider the psychological effects of extreme weight loss on themselves and those around them. It is not uncommon for couples to divorce or break up after this surgery. This chapter will help you understand what kind of emotions and roadblocks you may face in your relationships. Spouses or significant others often have similar reactions after bariatric surgery. What is described here is normal human behavior and is no reflection on the quality of your relationship or the character of your partner.

Before surgery, you have equilibrium in your relationship and in your home environment. After surgery, these things will change drastically. If you change, your partner has to change in some ways as well. People do not really enjoy change, especially when it is not their decision or their surgery. When this happens, the partner may attempt to change the relationship back to the way it was when it was familiar, comfortable, and he or she knew what to expect.

SABOTAGE

The actions taken by a partner to restore familiar equilibrium often take the form of sabotage to the diet and exercise program. Your partner may give a subtle sigh when you go to exercise or complain about not going to a restaurant or even bring you your favorite food "because I knew you'd love it." I have heard stories of wives that suddenly begin baking or cooking mouth-watering meals that their husbands cannot eat. Most do not even realize that they are doing it and are embarrassed when it is brought to their attention. If you notice this kind of behavior, talk to your partner. He or she is probably dealing with many feelings he or she does not feel comfortable expressing. A good conversation about how weight loss is affecting your family members usually helps.

We also show love with food. A person may cook for a spouse, but now continues to cook even after surgery because it is how she knows to show love. The husband may bring chocolates on Valentines Day, not meaning to sabotage but simply doing what he knows to do.

Another interesting family dynamic is one I never expected when I started working in this field. If a patient occupies the position of the largest person in the family, then loses weight, what family member now moves up to that position? I can guarantee they don't want that honor. Sabotage has taken place in this situation, and relationships have suffered. If a family member says, "I'm happy for your weight loss, just don't get smaller than I am," this could be a red flag.

THE ACTIONS TAKEN BY A PARTNER to restore familiar equilibrium often take the form of sabotage to the diet and exercise program.

COUPLES HAVING BARIATRIC SURGERY TOGETHER

It happens more and more often: Two people will have bariatric surgery together. It is difficult being the patient. It can also be trying for the significant other. When couples have the surgery together, it can be twice as hard. Each person has the problems of both the patient and the significant other. I have found that people in healthy relationships do well together, but those having problems often see increased relationship difficulties after surgery. If you plan to have the surgery with a partner, try to remain independent as far as exercise and food choices. Working out together is a bonus, but do not get into the habit of skipping workouts because your partner cannot participate. Do not let your partner be in charge of your habits.

Good communication is the key to a couple's success. Before the surgery, discuss the logistics of the changes you must make. After the surgery, talk to each other weekly about your feelings regarding the surgery and the changes you are both experiencing. It is possible to grow much closer as a couple as a result of this experience.

There will be a tendency to talk each other into tiny cheats. Typically, this is how it works: "C'mon, let's just have a little bit. We deserve it." Having the surgery together represents some increased challenges, but has the potential for increased excitement and support. Keep communication flowing and problems will be minimized.

✓ TO DO

There is a natural human tendency to want to try to put things back the way they were. This includes spouses and significant others. We are comfortable in our old habits. Often family members do not realize they have motives for bringing "cheat" foods into the house. Underneath the surface, they crave the old, comfortable habits of the past. If this occurs in your home, try having everyone talk about how they are doing with all the changes. Keeping the lines of communication open is the key. I recommend that my patients ask their significant others how they are doing every few weeks.

Often, there is a common fear underlying the sabotage. The spouse or partner feels that the patient is going to lose weight and leave him or her for someone else. This thinking may seem ridiculous, but chances are pretty good that your partner may have already joked about it. You may even joke that you will do it. The problem is that he or she is not really joking. It is a fear that drives people to sabotage their partners' efforts. If the lines of communication are closed, relationships are at a real risk of failing.

As you lose weight quickly after the surgery, it can be difficult to get used to your new body. It can be just as difficult for those around you. They may be very proud and happy for you, but they may also have a hard time adjusting to the changes. Bariatric surgery is almost as difficult for the family as it is for the patient.

OTHER REACTIONS FROM FAMILY MEMBERS... "LET ME JUST POINT OUT..."

Another common emotion felt by family members is fear that the patient will somehow hurt him- or herself. I hear, "She's not eating enough protein," and "He's not exercising," and "He's not chewing enough" or, "I feel uncomfortable eating in front of him" often from family members. The family member is usually very worried about the well being of the patient. He or she shows concern by constantly reminding the patient of what he or she should be doing. This constant friction can affect the relationship. I advise family members to make a serious effort not to do this. The patient has been through psychological assessment and is able to understand the requirements of diet and exercise. It will ultimately be up to him or her to take responsibility for his or her own behavior. Constant "reminding" only serves to alienate the patient and cause stress in the relationship. The relationship will improve if each person understands what the other is feeling and makes an effort to stop the behavior that aggravates the relationship.

AS YOU LOSE WEIGHT QUICKLY after the surgery, it can be difficult to get used to your new body. It can be just as difficult for those around you. They may be very proud and happy for you, but they may also have a hard time adjusting to the changes.

The best way for family to assist you in your efforts is to just be supportive, listen, and agree to keep those trigger foods out of the house. I always advise my patients not to put their spouses or families in the position of being the reminder, or the policeman. This puts them in a very difficult position, and when you do cheat, it can impact the relationship.

"YOU'RE TAKING THE EASY WAY OUT"

It is a natural tendency for people to attribute their own successes to intelligence, character, or hard work, and the successes of others to luck. So it is not uncommon to hear statements like, "He's taking the easy way out. He had bariatric surgery." This is, for the most part, a misguided attitude. People think it's easy because they are seduced by the drastic before and after pictures they see in the media. The truth is that almost everyone having bariatric surgery will lose weight, and lose it much more quickly than on any diet. This is the primary reason why so many think of it as the latest "I gotta try it" diet. I have met people who were only 65 pounds overweight, with no serious health problems, who actually tried to gain more weight so they would be eligible for the surgery. The surgery is often mistakenly viewed as the latest diet craze, or an easy, foolproof way to lose weight. It is the fastest way to lose weight, but it is anything but easy. Living with the aftermath of surgery may include sickness and unpleasant-looking physical changes. Your world as you know it will change, and you will be faced with having to exercise for the rest of your life. It is rare, but some people die from bariatric surgery, and others may end up with complications that land them back in the hospital again and again. The important thing to know is the psychology behind those who may try to talk you

Case Study

Theresa's family was very supportive of her weight loss. She weighed 400 pounds, and the rest of her family had body weights in the normal range. As she began to lose weight, she received much reinforcement from family members. After several months, her mother jokingly asked her to stop losing weight "before you get smaller than I am." This request was upsetting to her, and she brought it up in group therapy. The group members advised her to talk to her mother about it. She was afraid of alienating her mother with continued weight loss.

down. They may have struggled with their own weight and are looking to strike out at someone who has had tremendous success. Understand why they do it, and do not let it affect your success.

ANGER

Anger and resentment on the part of the family is a common occurrence at some point after surgery. The family is asked to make changes at home, worry about the life and health of the patient, and put up with some intense mood swings. As one of my patients explained, "It was my choice to have this surgery, but my family was drafted." The family may resent having to deal with the obesity issue in the first place. Even if they are supportive and loving, they may perceive that your obesity is due to a lack of prior action. I have heard patients' family members say, "This is unfair. I have been exercising all my life, but now I have to deal with this because he refused to exercise for 25 years. It is not right." This is a normal reaction and should pass with time. Encourage your family to tell you how they feel. If it does not improve, the problem runs deeper, and you should consider family counseling.

ABUSE

Some spouses will use weight as an excuse to abuse. They may make negative remarks, threaten to leave the relationship, withhold affection, and blame it all on the weight. This is considered emotional abuse. For some, it may even escalate to physical abuse. A person on the receiving end in this situation is likely to feel powerless, have low self esteem, and after weight loss, may decide to leave the relationship. If this describes you, leaving may be your best option. No one should endure physical or emotional abuse. At the very least, couples therapy should be undertaken.

OTHERS CONCERNED WITH YOUR WEIGHT

There are those mothers, fathers, or friends that have spent years telling you to lose weight. These are the ones that say, "Do you really think you should eat that extra helping?" They make comments about other people's weight around you and seem to have made it a hobby to point out your weight.

It is a strange phenomenon that when you do lose weight, often this same person starts to discuss how thin you are becoming or how you should "fatten up a little bit." For these people, it is difficult to stop talking about your weight because it has become a habit.

Well-meaning family members may also say things like, "You were so fat. You were gigantic. We all talked about it and didn't know what to do." They may

unwittingly say things that hurt your feelings. Discuss
their comments with them. They may not realize
what they are saying or how it makes you feel.

Your weight loss may change others' perceptions of
themselves. For example, if you are 5 feet 6 inches and
walk into a room full of professional basketball players,
you will perceive yourself as being short. If you walk
into a kindergarten classroom, you will feel tall. Your
weight loss will have psychological effects on those
around you as well as yourself.

Chapter **15**

Common Reactions to Weight Loss

There are many kinds of changes that can occur when one begins to lose weight after bariatric surgery. No one person experiences all of these changes, but most will encounter several of them.

"WHEN I LOOK IN A MIRROR I AM SHOCKED"

Almost everyone has this reaction to rapid weight loss. It takes time, and perhaps years, for your mental representation of yourself to match your new body dimensions. It is not uncommon to catch a glimpse of your reflection in a window or mirror and be shocked at what you see. When you are going about your daily business, your mind forgets what you have accomplished.

With time, you will come to terms with it. Some people adjust quickly, and others take years. Some may never have a realistic mental picture of themselves, especially if they spent most of their life being overweight. Even when overweight, people often do not have an accurate body image. Most recall shock at seeing photos of themselves and saying, "I didn't realize I had gained that much weight." Body image disparity is very common, especially in women.

There is both a physical and an emotional component to body image. The body changes rapidly, but the emotions change much more slowly. Expect it to take some time, even years. I advise my patients to think of it as a novelty. Your mental interpretation of the experience will play a part in determining if it is a minor annoyance or a major problem. If you interpret it as a minor annoyance, it will have less of an impact on you. Patience is the cure, and eventually your mental self will more closely coincide with your physical self.

> **THE BODY CHANGES RAPIDLY,** but the emotions change much more slowly.

One technique for learning to appreciate your true size/body image is to look at yourself in the mirror and find at least five things you like about your body. It could be your wrists, your calves, your neck, or even your fingers. Another technique is to look at photos of yourself at various stages of weight loss. Do not avoid the camera during this transition. It will help you stay in touch with your actual size. Take a photo once per month for the first year. Take it in the same place in your home, and these photos will help you to visualize your true size.

If you've only had a weight problem for a few years, you may not have a problem with body image. You may feel you are simply returning to your old self. If you've had a weight problem for many years, especially if you started to gain weight as a child, the person looking back in the mirror may feel like a stranger.

If for some reason your body image disparity does not resolve on its own, it may be necessary to attend some groups, talk to other patients, or talk to a psychologist about the problem. The negative messages some people receive throughout their lives do not magically dissipate after weight loss and can interfere with having a more accurate body image.

FEELING CONFIDENT

With confidence, you can walk into a room without feeling as though people think you are fat. You will feel free to be yourself without worrying about how you look. This newfound feeling may translate into taking more chances with your life. Perhaps you will find new relationships, a new career, a new sport, or other new challenges. Your confidence will increase with each success as you learn to take control. You begin to replace "I can't" with "I can." Confidence is a wonderful feeling, and your assignment is to enjoy it. Use it to achieve your goals, whatever they may be.

FEELINGS OF ACCOMPLISHMENT

You did it! You have been through so much and you are winning! Other problems may appear smaller by comparison. This feeling helps keep you motivated to continue with your diet and exercise program. Perhaps you have been setting goals and achieving rewards. This serves to increase your feeling of accomplishment.

There are no expected ways to behave or change after bariatric surgery. Do not feel pressured to make sweeping changes in your life to live up to other people's expectations. Be kind to yourself and move at your own pace. But do not be surprised if after your recent success, you choose to tackle other issues in your life.

FEELING NORMAL

For the first time in ages, your weight is in the normal range and you feel less self-conscious. You feel like you fit in. You can shop in regular stores in the mall, and others can buy clothes for you. You can fit into rides at theme parks and in airplane seats. Your weight no longer sets you apart, and this feeling can be comforting and exhilarating. Congratulations!

FEELING LESS HELPLESS

After trying one diet after another, many people begin to feel helpless over their weight. Over time, that feeling of helplessness can expand to other areas of your life, such as career, relationships, health, or even your future. Another effect of weight loss is feeling an increased sense of control and a decreased sense of helplessness. This is an empowering feeling as you realize your future is in your own hands. Again, enjoy the feeling. Feeling in control is a powerful emotion that can open up a world of opportunities for you.

FOCUSING ON OTHER PEOPLE'S WEIGHT

You've seen it many times. The ex-smoker who can't stop talking about smoking or pointing out other people's smoking. They may dramatically gag and cough at the sight of a smoker. A similar fixation can also occur in people who lose a large amount of weight. The formerly overweight person becomes obsessed with other people's weight and urges others to do what they did. They may even comment on overweight people they see or offer "well-meaning" advice just as others did to them. This person is excited about all the changes he or she has made, and it seems that all he or she can talk about is weight loss. On the other hand, this behavior can be distasteful and disturbing to others around him or her and can even serve to alienate old friends.

FEELING IN CONTROL is a powerful emotion that can open up a world of opportunities for you.

Excitement about your success is a good thing, but monitor yourself and be aware of the reactions of others. If you have a tendency to be this way, be aware that many an old friendship have disintegrated due to this kind of obsession.

"MY FRIENDS ARE JEALOUS OF MY WEIGHT LOSS"

The possibility exists that some people will be jealous of your weight loss, especially if you previously enjoyed eating out together or dining at each other's homes. You may all have enjoyed food without having thought about its connection to weight. Perhaps the subject of weight was ignored because you were all in the same boat. But now you have not only changed the dynamic of the group, you have shined a light on the subject of weight. These friends may now feel uncomfortable around you because you have succeeded, especially if they have attempted weight loss themselves. Talk to them about how you feel, and listen openly to their feelings. Voicing your concerns can begin to alleviate them, or in some situations, it just takes time for them to get used to the changes. It is your right to discuss anything you like, but try to keep the conversation on subjects you enjoyed prior to

Case Study

Stephanie did very well after bariatric surgery. One year after the surgery, she had lost more than 150 pounds. She went to the gym almost every day. She was truly a success story. One day I received a frantic phone call. She was angry and said, "All of my friends are jealous of my weight loss." She complained that she was not being invited to activities because of this jealousy. We talked for a while, and it became apparent that she was engaging in certain behaviors that were driving her friends away. She was urging them all to lose weight, and they felt uncomfortable being around their friend because of her inability to discuss subjects other than food or weight. Going out to dinner as they had in the past had become a trying experience for everyone. We came up with a plan. She understood that it was her enthusiasm that was exciting and motivating her to talk about weight and weight loss, but that perhaps it was uncomfortable for those around her to hear. She decided to try to change her interactions with her friends to include subjects other than food and weight loss, and she called several weeks later to say that her relationships with her friends had indeed improved, and they had not been jealous, just bored and uncomfortable.

Now and then Stephanie comes to a support group. She says her relationships are doing well, and she often counsels others in the group to watch their conversations with friends.

weight loss. There will be fewer problems if everyone involved feels as though nothing has really changed.

CHANGING YOUR LIFE

Rapid weight loss can be exciting. The first year or so after the surgery can be life-changing. Not only are you changing physically, but you are changing emotionally as well. Emotions tend to be very strong that first year, and people sometimes get caught up in the excitement. I recommend not making any major life changes during this first year. Give your emotions time to reach an equilibrium. Try to focus on your health and habits for the first year, and save the big decisions, such as marriage, divorce, or having children, for several months down the road.

CHANGING YOUR STYLE OF DRESS

Admit it. You have dreamed about it, fantasized about it, and you are ready to wear what you want and have fun with your clothes. You may find your style of dress has completely changed, often becoming a bit more trendy or more provocative. The thought of being able to wear what we want often helps to keep us on our diet and exercise program. However, some people take it to the extreme. I sometimes get calls from family members who complain, "She's gone off the deep end and wears tube tops and mini skirts." Whatever your clothing choice, be aware that others are watching you and may be concerned with the changes. Consider talking about it with those who have difficulty with the "new you." Your clothing choice is yours alone to make, and you deserve to enjoy yourself after all your hard work.

At the other end of the spectrum, some feel there must be something wrong with them because they do not want to wear tight-fitting clothes. They feel more comfortable in loose fitting clothes. This too is normal. Try not to let others' expectations influence your choices. There is no right or wrong way to dress. What is right for you is right.

"I'M THIN, BUT I STILL FEEL DIFFERENT THAN OTHER PEOPLE"

You may feel "different" for some time. After all, you are different. You have a tiny stomach and do not have the same food choices you had in the past. You have gone through drastic lifestyle, physical, and psychological changes. Yes, you are different, but that will be a positive or negative depending on your perspective.

✓ TO DO

1. Tell yourself it is OK to feel like you are different.
2. Concentrate on the positives and everything you have gained.
3. Ask yourself, "Am I better off now than I was before?"

FEAR OF WEIGHT GAIN

A large percentage of patients experience an intense fear of regaining their weight. For many, they have experienced what they consider to be a miracle. Often, after a lifelong battle with weight, they have won, but the nagging question is, "How long will I be able to keep it off?" This feeling is normal when you think about the yo-yo dieting that most patients have gone through. History tells us that excitement over weight loss is almost always replaced by sadness and disgust over weight gain. It is no wonder we fear the return of weight, even after bariatric surgery.

If you follow the diet and continue to exercise for life, you will most likely not gain the weight back. You should expect to gain a little back eventually. This is considered normal. But if you follow the diet and continue to exercise for life, you should feel confident that you can keep it off. Let the knowledge that you and only you have the power to keep it off and be a motivator to stick with it. Even with this knowledge, some people will react in an unhealthy way. Here are a few examples:

Hypervigilance. This reaction is one of precision. If a person is supposed to eat two ounces of chicken, then they make absolutely sure they are not eating 2.1 ounces. A patient of mine would focus on eating the exact amount of food she was allotted, and not one bit more. Going over the allotted amount would cause a very negative effect. She would become sad,

Case Study

Lina had been overweight all her life. Before surgery she said, "I can't imagine what it will be like when I actually have a normal weight." After surgery, she lost more than 120 pounds in about six months. She was excited, people were relating to her in a completely different way, and she lost perspective. Although she had been married for more than 20 years, she met a man on the Internet, and sight unseen, moved to Italy to live with him. She would not be talked out of it or convinced to wait. About five months later she returned, and wanted her old life back again—now that she had a more realistic perspective. She was luckily able to reestablish the relationship with her husband, but not all spouses are that understanding. It is always a good idea to give drastic changes some time.

withdrawn, guilty, and anxious. She would follow this with an extra 45-minute workout to "compensate" for the lapse.

Over time, this reaction tends to become more extreme. Not only is it difficult to be so precise, but it can drive others crazy. Also, it makes very little difference in overall weight loss and weight maintenance. As with other psychological reactions, the first step is becoming aware of the behavior. The next step is to attempt to change it. If you are unable to change the behavior on your own, seek help from a psychologist for a few weeks to overcome the reaction. A trained professional can usually help you to get the behavior under control fairly quickly.

Obsessing over five pounds. Weight maintenance is not a horizontal line on a graph. A person's weight will be up and down 5, 10, 15, 20 pounds multiple times over the course of their lifetime. Most patients will develop a weight range in which they feel comfortable. When this range is exceeded, it can trigger a list of behaviors that will bring the weight down to an acceptable level. Body weight changes in response to many factors, and can vary 5 to 10 pounds just with water retention. Some patients obsess about this, having a good day with no gain, and a bad day if they're up a pound or two. Try to look at the big picture. Weight will fluctuate. Don't allow the number on the scale to dictate mood. Merely make a couple of adjustments to your behavior in response to the number, and the weight should drop back into your comfort range.

Purging. Purging is self-induced vomiting. There are people with no history of purging who suddenly start after surgery. The root of this problem is fear of

Case Study

Charlotte had unrealistic hopes for the surgery. She thought she would not be tempted to eat her favorite foods, or, if she did, she would be satisfied with a bite or two. Unfortunately, she soon found she battled the same urges to eat she had always experienced in the past. She was unable to stop herself from eating the foods she has always loved, and discovered that she could "undo the damage" by purging. Charlotte had never used purging as a means to control weight prior to surgery. She admitted this in a monthly support group for bariatric patients.

She told me it started because she felt she had too much to lose if she ate what she liked, so she purged. She said, "I never lost this much weight before, and I'm so scared of going backward again." This behavior is very difficult to stop, and the health ramifications can be catastrophic. It took months of very hard work in therapy to solve the problem.

weight gain, coupled with an inability to control emotional eating patterns.

Purging is a full-fledged eating disorder. If you have never purged, do not try it. If you are now purging, you are putting your health in serious jeopardy and must stop immediately. Ask for professional help if you are unable to stop on your own.

Take note of these warning signs. If you are in the habit of taking a bite, chewing it up, then spitting it out, you could be taking the first steps toward a dangerous eating disorder. It may eventually progress to swallowing and purging. If you know that the next bite will make you vomit, but you take it anyway, that is an eating disorder. I've heard patients say "I didn't put my finger down my throat, so it's not an eating disorder."

Without getting too graphic, as a bariatric patient you probably won't have to do that. An eating disorder is just as devastating to your health and well being as obesity, so don't fool yourself.

Eating too few calories for good health. This reaction is one of "if a little is good, then even less will be better." You will already be highly restricted in the amount of calories per day you are able to consume. A person with this reaction will start to eat even less. It is not a hard habit to get into since you already will not be very hungry. Less is not more in the case of bariatric patients. It is difficult to get enough nutrition after surgery, but restricting it even further can have very negative effects on your health.

If you find yourself in this category, know that the longer you continue the behavior, the more difficult it will be to stop. Know also that weight loss after surgery is rapid even with the recommended diet. If you are unable to stop on your own, seek the help of a professional as soon as possible. This is the equivalent of an eating disorder and can be dangerous to your health.

Often, it is the family that brings this problem to the attention of the patient. They worry about the amount of food intake and possibly the unhealthy physical appearance of the patient and decide confrontation is the answer. You may not even realize there is a problem until confronted. If this happens, please listen to their concerns, and realize your perspective on food might not be realistic.

This surgery requires a change in perspective about dieting. On regular diets, the thinking is the less you eat, the more you lose. After bariatric surgery, the thinking must change to "I'll lose quickly and remain healthy by filling my pouch with

Case Study

Stephanie lost more than 100 pounds with the surgery, and ended up being a size 10. As a business executive, she said she had always been considered "competent and intelligent," but after her weight loss, she was considered "a piece of meat" by the men in the company. She was highly disturbed by this change in reaction of men, and looked for reasons to avoid interactions with men outside of work. Weight can allow a person to be sexually invisible for the most part. Weight loss may take away the sexual barrier and may be uncomfortable to some patients.

high-quality proteins." Rapid weight loss without following your prescribed diet is not healthy, and it is possible to end up back in the hospital with complications. You now require the high-octane food your body craves. Nourish it well. Follow the program guidelines and you will lose the weight.

OBSESSION OVER THE BODY

Many people have plastic surgery after they lose weight. For some, they have significant amounts of hanging skin and surgery is necessary for them to be able to function in their day-to-day lives. Others have it for less pressing reasons. Some patients become obsessed with their outward appearance and have multiple plastic surgeries.

An interesting change often happens like this: A person loses weight, starts to buy more stylish clothes, perhaps even starts a new life. The positive feedback from self or others can be like a drug. There is some research that suggests when a person has plastic surgery he or she becomes less satisfied with other parts of the body, leading to more and more procedures. A person obsessed with plastic surgery may have only been concerned with the inner person before surgery, but afterward became fixated on the superficial aspects of the outer person.

Plastic surgery is necessary for many people after a bariatric procedure, but it can become a dangerous obsession. There is a fine line between elective surgery and obsession. Plastic surgery can increase self esteem and decrease physical problems associated with excess skin, and in most cases, patients are pleased with the results. Each surgery carries a risk, however, and requires a considerable amount of careful planning and good judgment.

Case Study

Jessica lost 225 pounds after her bypass and was ecstatic. Once her weight stabilized, she had a series of plastic surgeries on her abdomen, her buttocks, and her upper arms. She looked great. The following year she had her neck, breasts, and eyes done. She came to the group to discuss her plastic surgeries and how she was feeling. She mentioned she was saving to have a facelift next and described plastic surgery as "fun." One of the other patients in the group asked her what had happened to her. The person he knew was easy going, down to earth, and comfortable in her own skin. This new Jessica was obsessed with outward physical details. He said this new person was a stranger. She became upset, and did not come back to the group. She was not willing to hear any feedback about it.

"WHY DO I FEEL ANGER?"

Patients do not usually expect to feel angry a couple of months after surgery, but it is more common than most people think. Let's face it— overweight people often are treated badly in our society. They are called names, pointed at, laughed at, discriminated against, and, as a result, usually have low self-esteem because of this. There seems to be a perception in the general population that weight loss surgery is an "easy out," and prejudice against overweight people in our society is still accepted. Unfortunately, if you hear that obese people are lazy, unmotivated, and have no willpower, over time you are likely to start believing these labels yourself.

When someone is disrespectful to you as an obese person, you may be angry and may even come to expect it. When you lose weight, people may begin to treat you differently. You may be treated with more respect. This may unexpectedly bring out feelings of anger in some patients because you are still the same person you always were. The only thing that has changed is the outside. Patients tell me, "I should be happy someone whistled at me today, but instead I just feel sad and angry."

This is only a stage in your weight loss journey, and you will pass through it. Be patient with yourself and be patient with people in general. Again, it is human nature to judge a book by its cover to some extent. You are just sporting a new cover. My patients tell me it is a phase, and eventually you will become more accepting of the reactions of others. The challenge is not to isolate yourself or withdraw from others because of this feeling.

The bottom line is that others' perceptions of us have an effect on how we see ourselves. Just as the label of "lazy" has an effect when one is obese, the label of "piece of meat" can have an effect as well. Never forget that your personality, your qualities, and your value as a human being remain no matter what size you are.

RETURN TO OLD HABITS TO PLEASE OTHERS

Many patients have sad stories from their past. Maybe they include a dominating family member who rejects them after weight loss. There may be a subconscious urge to regain weight in order to regain acceptance with this person. This is a dangerous situation and should be handled in individual therapy. Often, the patient does not know why he or she is regaining the weight. It is not a problem with your weight that alienates you from the person, but a problem within that person. Thankfully, this is not a very common occurrence, but it is serious and requires professional help.

"I CAN'T BE FINISHED LOSING ALL THE WEIGHT"

It is not uncommon to hear a patient say, "The doctor told me I am at goal weight, but I think he's wrong." There is so much positive reinforcement from weight loss that it is often difficult to admit you have achieved the goal after years of trying. The reluctance or inability to accept that the maintenance stage has been reached is extremely difficult for some patients. Some people will say "I've achieved my goal weight, but I still need to lose five more pounds." A person may spend years trying to lose weight and then more time getting the surgery and going through everything involved. When your goal weight is finally achieved, it can be difficult after that tremendous effort to shift your focus to something else. Weight loss can become like a drug, and the reactions of others can become addicting.

COME TO TERMS with the fact that thinking about weight loss has been an all-consuming passion, but that now it is time to look beyond the weight.

✓ TO DO

Come to terms with the fact that thinking about weight loss has been an all-consuming passion, but that now it is time to look beyond the weight. It is OK to add some foods back into your diet. You did it! It is time to enjoy all those things you had in mind when you went for the surgery. Your job will never be completely finished though, because you must still concentrate on the maintenance of lifelong exercise and a healthy diet. This is a time to test different foods and explore your new mobility and outlook. You have earned the right to enjoy yourself.

The most important thing to remember about all of these possible emotional changes is to keep the lines of communication open with your friends, family, and coworkers. Do not be afraid to enlist the help of a professional when necessary. Welcome and encourage feedback about the new you. You can learn from each other if you keep an open mind.

"MY SURGERY DIDN'T WORK"

Unrealistic expectations are not uncommon. I've heard many patients say, "My surgery didn't work. I can still eat anything I want." People who have the expectation that surgery will stop them from eating will be disappointed. Surgery will never cure an eating disorder and will not stop a person from eating long term. It is so important for bariatric patients to receive proper education and to have realistic expectations. If you think you are not getting all the information you need from your program, contact your program's coordinator. You should feel comfortable that you have all the tools you need for success. This includes realistic expectations and information about your future.

"I THOUGHT ALL MY PROBLEMS WOULD GO AWAY AFTER I LOST WEIGHT"

It is easy to look at before and after photos and think, "She sure seems happy. No problems can be big problems when you look like that." Realistically, people have problems no matter what they weigh. Whether it be relationship conflicts, bills, health issues, anxiety, or anything else, weight loss is not the answer. People who magically expect happiness with weight loss are often shocked and disappointed that many of their problems still exist.

This can be a difficult time for some patients. It is easy to attribute almost all of our problems to weight before surgery, but to what do we attribute them after weight loss? Losing weight can provide many incredible benefits, but guaranteed happiness is not one of them. If you are in this category, it would be very helpful to go to therapy for a few months. With the help of a psychologist and/or some support groups, you can work toward sorting out your problems and hopefully finding some of that elusive happiness.

Depression After Surgery

L ife after bariatric surgery will be different. How it differs will vary from person to person. Some patients will become depressed after surgery. This section will help you learn to identify symptoms of depression and how to help yourself. You might say, "I can't imagine being depressed when losing weight." Believe it or not, this happens frequently. When people go through surgery and/or drastic lifestyle changes, depression can be a side effect. I have seen patients who previously had a tendency to become depressed react to the stress of surgery by falling into a depressive episode.

HOW DO I KNOW IF I'M DEPRESSED?

The majority of bariatric patients will not become depressed following surgery. For others, however, depression can range from mild to severe. It is important to be able to recognize the symptoms of depression, so you may ask for help if needed.

About one-third of patients report some minor symptoms of depression. We refer to this as "post-op blues." People will say the overriding thought is "Why did I do this? What was I thinking?" The adjustment period may be difficult. Your body will be living off stored energy, which can make patients feel tired and lethargic. This is not true depression, and will usually go away on its own in a couple of months. It is normal to feel this way. It's usually nothing to worry about unless it gets worse.

Symptoms of depression:

1. **Sadness.** A depressed person does not have to be sad all the time. Feeling sad most of the time or most of the days per week is enough.

2. **Loss of interest.** A depressed person does not look forward to events or activities anymore. This person may have liked going to the theater for example, but now it sounds like more trouble than it is worth.

3. **Changes in sleep habits.** A depressed person may feel very tired and sleep more hours than usual, or may find him- or herself sleeping less than usual. For example, this person may find it difficult to get to sleep, and then wake up very early in the morning without being able to go back to sleep. Sleep apnea can influence your answer to this question.

4. **Changes in appetite.** For some, food may not look appetizing and food intake will decrease. For others, hunger is a constant and they will be more focused on food. It is not uncommon for a person to gain weight from an increased appetite due to depression and then blame the depression on the weight gain. For these people, treatment usually results in weight loss. Bariatric surgery may influence this symptom because you may not feel hungry.

5. **Social isolation.** You may look for reasons to stay home and not see your friends. You may cancel activities with others because of a headache or tell them you have to do a chore. When a person is depressed, her world will shrink. She often sees fewer people, engages in fewer activities, and spends more time alone at home. This just serves to increase the depression.

6. **Helplessness.** A depressed person will begin to feel that he has no control over the events in his life. He often feels like a victim, and that there is no action he can take that will alleviate the pain and suffering or fix the problem.

7. **Hopelessness.** Often a depressed person will feel as though there is no hope for the future, or she can't see herself ever feeling better. To her, it seems like sadness will follow her forever.

8. **Worthlessness.** Some people talk about the overwhelming feeling of worthlessness that sometimes accompanies depression. It is common for this person to isolate further and ignore offers

from others for help. He is, after all, "not worth the trouble."

9. **Irritability.** Usually a depressed person will feel more irritable and easily angered. She may be quick to jump to negative conclusions about others. A family member may be the first to bring it to her attention, but an irritable person may not be ready to hear this news.

10. **Low motivation.** A depressed person may find it difficult to get through his "to do" list for the day. He may have to force himself to take care of his usual chores, routines, self care, and activities.

11. **Suicidal ideation.** This is the most dangerous symptom of all. If you are contemplating suicide or have said to yourself, "Things would be better if I wasn't around," then your situation is extreme. It is imperative that you get help immediately. Research that came out in the fall of 2007 showed an elevated suicide rate in patients after bariatric surgery, 5 to 8 times higher than people who have not had bariatric surgery. It is important to note that suicide is not a side effect of bariatric surgery, but there does appear to be a vulnerability. Each person having the surgery should be aware of this research so they can monitor their own symptoms and ask for help if needed. Never take chances. If you are thinking about suicide, this is very serious. When one is depressed, suicide can seem like a solution, but it is the depression itself that causes this skewed

thinking. I have worked with many patients that became suicidal, but months later when the depression was alleviated, they said, "Thank goodness I didn't do it. It seemed like a way out at the time." If this describes you, you must call for help immediately. Talk to a family member, call a professional, or call 911 if it is an emergency. You do not have to feel depressed. There is help.

If you have several of the symptoms listed above, it is important to get help, especially if it is affecting your work or relationships. Depression can be alleviated. Without treatment, most depression will usually decrease on its own in about six months, but do not wait. Untreated depression makes it difficult to stick to lifestyle changes and may lead to problems with weight loss or maintenance. Get the professional help you need as soon as you realize you have a problem.

With the assistance of professionals, depression can be decreased or even alleviated in weeks or a short period of time. State-of-the-art treatment for

WITHOUT TREATMENT, most depression will usually decrease on its own in about six months, but do not wait. Untreated depression makes it difficult to stick to lifestyle changes and may lead to problems with weight loss or maintenance.

depression involves both antidepressants and talk therapy. Research continues to show that these two treatments together are the best and fastest way to decrease depressive symptoms. The most important advice is to see a professional if you feel depressed. There is help.

For a prescription for an antidepressant, you may seek the expertise of a psychiatrist. The psychiatrist will prescribe the antidepressant that is most useful for people with symptoms similar to yours. Not all psychiatrists perform psychotherapy. Some patients

> **WHEN ONE IS DEPRESSED,** suicide may seem like a solution, but it is the depression itself that causes this skewed thinking.

prefer to use their PCPs (primary care physicians) to prescribe an antidepressant, but some PCPs are reluctant to do this. Whichever route you choose, understand that antidepressants take from 3 to 6 weeks to work, and there will be side effects. Discuss the specifics with the doctor that prescribed them for you.

For talk therapy, you should seek the expertise of a psychologist, psychiatrist who performs psychotherapy, social worker, or mental health counselor. You should likely do what is called cognitive-behavioral therapy. This treatment works with your thought patterns and behaviors to alleviate depression and has been shown in research to work well.

Depression can come from many different sources. Some of these sources are the following:

1. **Mourning the loss of food.** Food has always been there as a way to help you cope with emotions. After bariatric surgery, you may feel like you are on the outside looking in, especially when socializing or in restaurants. This mourning period is normal and will usually subside with time.

2. **Depression can come from the reactions you receive from family, coworkers, spouses, and even strangers.** The reactions of others may be positive or negative, but the change itself may lead to depression as you begin to alter your self image.

3. **Those who have a history of depression may become depressed due to the stress of life after surgery.** Patients with a history of depression should have a psychologist they can see after surgery to be monitored for any increase in symptoms.

4. **Those who had unrealistic expectations that weight loss would make them happy are at risk for depression.**

5. **It is common for people focused on weight to base their mood on the number on the scale.** If the number on the scale is up, mood becomes depressed. If the number on the scale goes down, mood becomes happy. Do not fall into that trap. Weight will normally fluctuate depending on many

physical factors throughout the day, week, or month. Do not let your mood be dictated by a number on the scale. I recommend choosing a range based on your goal and normal fluctuations. For example, if your weight goal is 150, choose a realistic weight range of 150 to 160. Weigh yourself weekly. As long as your weight stays within this range, you are OK. If it exceeds this range, you need to make some changes. Refer to the Emergency First Aid section in this book, if necessary.

6. **The surgery itself may be a trigger for an episode of depression.** It is more of a biological reaction to the surgery rather than a logical reaction. This type can be compared to postpartum depression, where a person can be thrilled to have a new baby, but become depressed against all logic.

ANTIDEPRESSANTS, ANTIPSYCHOTICS, MOOD STABILIZERS, AND ANTIANXIETY MEDICATIONS

There are many medicines that are critical for some patients to maintain functioning in their daily lives, including antidepressants, antipsychotics, mood stabilizers, and anxiolytics. After bariatric surgery, it will be difficult, if not impossible, to take pills for some time. Therefore, it is extremely important to check with your prescriber before surgery about how you can take the medication after surgery. Some medication can be crushed and mixed with yogurt. Some can be prescribed in liquid form. Some even come in strips that dissolve on the tongue or as long-term injectables. It is critical that the medication not be stopped as this may lead to major mental health problems. Inform your surgeon about your psychotropic medications so they can resume them in the hospital, and then continue with them when you arrive home. Never stop your medication without medical supervision as this may trigger an episode. The dose may have to be adjusted depending on weight loss or absorption issues. If depression stems from weight gain, it will likely be alleviated with weight loss. However, weight loss will never cure bipolar disorder, schizophrenia, some depression, or multiple other mental health problems that may need medication to control.

MENTAL ILLNESS AND BARIATRIC SURGERY

"If I have been diagnosed with a mental illness, can I still have bariatric surgery?" The answer is generally yes, but with added precautions. Being diagnosed with a mental illness is not a rule-out for bariatric surgery, but it does mean some additional planning will be necessary to assist the patient after surgery.

SAFETY NET

Patients have had bariatric surgery after being diagnosed with depression, bipolar disorder, anxiety disorder, or schizophrenia. A patient who has a history of mental illness should make sure he or she has a safety net in place for the very stressful postoperative period. For example, if a person has a history of major depression, he or she is at risk for depression after surgery. In that case, a safety net of a psychologist and/or a psychiatrist that can frequently meet with the patient after surgery is necessary. If symptoms increase, the professional will see it early and help to reduce symptoms.

A person with mental illness has special considerations that should be addressed before he or she has bariatric surgery. A general guideline is that you should be functioning normally for a period of time and feel that your medication is working well for you before considering bariatric surgery. Because the postoperative period tends to be stressful and emotions change rapidly after surgery, it is not advisable to consider surgery until this guideline has been met.

Certain mental illnesses occur at a higher rate in people who are obese. These include depression, anxiety, and posttraumatic stress disorder. We have a chicken and egg problem here because we don't yet know if some mental illness causes obesity or is a result of obesity. Interestingly, years after surgery about half of patients with certain mental illnesses before surgery say they have experienced improvement in symptoms.

Surgery will not cure all depression. Approximately 20 percent of surgery patients are depressed before surgery. For many of these, depression will not diminish, or it may for a period of time but then return after weight loss. For some, it will be completely alleviated. I had a patient ask me if weight loss would cure her bipolar disorder. It appears to be a commonly held belief that surgery and weight loss will cure mental illness, but it is absolutely not the case.

If you have a mental illness, especially if you've been an inpatient in a psychiatric hospital or have ever attempted or thought of suicide, please disclose all of this information during your psychiatric evaluation. Your psychologist will ask you about it, and he or she can then establish a safety net for you.

Especially in light of the higher suicide rate after surgery, it is very important to be honest with your evaluator. Safety is the primary concern here.

✓ TO DO

1. Psychiatric medication, such as antidepressants and antipsychotics, are very important during the postoperative period. Do not make any major changes to your medication regimen if it is working.

2. The person prescribing your psychotropic medications can also make recommendations about the medication after surgery since you won't be able to take pills for some time. Find out beforehand if your medication can be crushed and mixed with yogurt, or if an oral liquid or injectable form of the drug can be prescribed.

3. Your mental health providers need to be aware of your surgery. Be sure they are available to see you after surgery to monitor for problems.

4. After a malabsorptive procedure there may be changes in the way certain medicines are absorbed. Check with the person who prescribes your medicine about how you should handle this. They can be a good resource after surgery and can provide information on absorption issues and how to take your medicine.

5. Always tell your surgeon about any antidepressant, mood stabilizer, or antipsychotic medication you may be taking so it can be prescribed in the hospital. As soon as you get home, get right back on your medication regimen. Never stop taking a psychotropic medication without supervision.

Is It True That Some People Do Not Lose Very Much Weight After Surgery?

There are several categories of patients who may experience some psychological problems related to food after surgery. Listed in the upcoming pages are some of the problems that have been reported. If any of these apply to you, you should make an appointment as soon as possible with a psychologist by calling the 800 number on the back of your insurance card or consulting with your bariatric program's psychologist. Most of these problems can be helped if professionals are consulted early.

THE UNCONTROLLED EMOTIONAL EATER

This person has not addressed the reasons why he eats and consumes food "automatically" out of habit or when bored, stressed, or sad. The first six months after surgery, a person may lose weight, even while eating in this way, but eventually the weight loss will stop and he or she will begin to gain it back. If he or she is in a bariatric support group, he or she will realize others are losing weight and he or she is not losing as much. Everyone I speak to before the surgery is convinced they will be able to handle the drastic change in a lifelong pattern of eating behavior, but unfortunately this is not always the case. If you see yourself in this scenario, please contact a psychologist. In sessions, you will examine thoughts and triggers that are associated with this emotional eating, and you will learn many techniques to put you back in control.

THE VICTIM OF ABUSE

Too many people in our society are sexually, physically, and/or emotionally abused as children. A traumatic past can have an effect on a person's life for many years, even if he or she is unaware of the impact. For a small percentage of victims, weight serves the unconscious purpose of protection. It is usually a feeling as opposed to an articulated thought, but it can affect a patient's ability to lose weight after surgery. These victims may subconsciously use weight to feel tougher, to make themselves unattractive, to avoid attention, or to keep people at a physical or emotional distance. It is not unusual for a victim of abuse to experience a drastic slowdown in weight loss several months after surgery. They report experiencing feelings of vulnerability, anxiety, feeling exposed, or feeling unsafe. The usual psychological reaction is to eat a little bit too much, so weight loss stops, and the uncomfortable feelings cease. This is understandable behavior under the circumstances. It is extremely uncomfortable and frightening for someone to lose that safety cocoon.

If you have an abuse history, it does not mean you will experience this. It is not a universal reaction to abuse, and there are multiple reasons why a person has a weight problem. But if you notice you have a couple of months with no significant weight loss, this may be a reason.

These feelings can be controlled, but therapy is required. In therapy, you can learn to deal with the anxiety caused by the weight loss. Within several weeks, most people are feeling stronger, in control, and are then able to continue with the program.

THE BINGE EATER

Binge eating can be understood as eating more food than most people would eat in a certain amount of time or in a certain situation. The most important aspect to binge eating is the feeling of being out of control. Binge eaters do not necessarily make themselves vomit after eating. There is usually a feeling of shame, guilt, or disgust after binging.

Binge eating is considered a risky behavior. If you binge before surgery, you will likely experience an urge to binge after surgery. Stress, difficult relationships, life changes, and even dieting can lead to an increase in episodes. After surgery, it is difficult to eat large quantities, so some people become frequent snackers or "grazers."

Binging is considered an eating disorder. Binging/grazing has been associated with weight regain after surgery, so it is important to learn to control this behavior. An eating disorder specialist can help you. Choose a psychologist familiar with eating disorders. You may also be directed to a psychiatrist for an evaluation for an antidepressant.

Case Study

Joshua had a problem with binge eating. At the age of 28, he had been binging for five years. When his weight reached 300 pounds, he decided to have bariatric surgery. At his presurgery psychological appointment, he did not disclose that he was binging, and his surgery was scheduled. Two years later, after reaching 175 pounds, he began to regain weight. When his weight reached 240 pounds, he came to my office for help.

It took almost six months of weekly therapy and hard work for Joshua to gain control over his eating. He said he was embarrassed by the binging, did most of his eating in secret, and did not want to tell anyone before the surgery. He was certain that the surgery would "cure" him of the problem. He said, "I thought because I would be losing weight I would be motivated to stop, but it didn't work."

Joshua checks in every now and then. He told me binging is still an issue, but he wins most of the time. He has been able to maintain a weight of 200 pounds for more than a year.

Binge eating is treatable and controllable with help. Start with a group and/or individual therapy. Only you know if you feel out of control with your eating, so if necessary, please ask for assistance.

THE UNREALISTIC PATIENT

Some people come into bariatric surgery with the expectation that it will magically force them to rigidly follow a diet. If they have been unable to follow a diet in the past, they may also have difficulty after surgery. These people may decide that it does not matter if they follow the diet because they have the same impulses to cheat that they have always had. At some point, they regret having the surgery and may start eating more than they should, which in turn stretches out the pouch.

Again, the best action is to contact a psychologist as soon as possible, before irreversible damage has been done to the pouch. With serious effort, you can learn to be in control of your food rather than the food being in control of you.

Case Study

Alberto had his jaw wired shut 20 years ago. He lost to his goal weight, but as soon as the wires were removed he went right back to his old eating habits and regained all the weight. Ten years ago, he had a bariatric procedure. Again, he lost the weight, but regained it all within two years. Alberto was always looking for something external (surgery, wires) to stop him from eating. He came to me wanting another bariatric surgery. From his history, it was clear he would need help in order to be successful with keeping the weight off. Alberto came to therapy for three months, during which time he focused on all the thoughts, behaviors, and excuses he had used most of his life. With practice, and by learning to control anxiety and stress, he began to stop himself from eating, rather than expecting something external to stop him. He had his surgery, and now has kept the weight off for more than three years. The surgery will work short term, but it will not work long term without the patient also learning to use the mind. If you are looking for something, other than you, to stop you from eating, weight loss will be short lived. For Alberto, it meant he had to focus on diet and exercise for the rest of his life. This time he has the psychological tools to help him accomplish his goals.

Afterword

With the decision to have bariatric surgery, you have also decided to take back control of your health. After weight loss, your future looks brighter, your health improves, and your choices in life increase. Hopefully, the information in this book will help you with the daunting task of maintaining your weight loss for life. For some patients, maintenance will be a breeze and habits will become automatic. For others, it will be a lifelong struggle, but one that can be won. Remember to always ask for help if you need it. The quest for a healthy life will never end, but the benefits and rewards definitely "outweigh" the challenge.

Resources

Academy for Eating Disorders. 6728 Old McLean Village Drive, McLean, VA 22101 www.aedweb.org.

Adami GF, Meneghelli A, Bressani A, Scopinaro, N. Body image in obese patients before and after stable weight reduction following bariatric surgery. *Journal of Psychosomatic Research* 1999;46(3):275–81.

Adolfsson B, Andersson I, Elofsson S, et al. Locus of control and weight reduction. *Patient Education and Counseling* 2005;56(1):55–61.

Alexander C. Depression after bariatric surgery: triggers, identification, treatment and prevention. *Bariatric Times.* 2008;5(5):24–6.

Alexander C. Psychological challenges influencing weight maintenance after bariatric surgery. *General Surgery News* (Obesity Care Special Edition). 2007;June: 59–63.

American College of Sports Medicine. (ACSM) P.O. Box,1440, Indianapolis, IN 46206 www.acsm.org/index.asp.

American Psychiatric Association. *Diagnostic and Statistical Manual on Mental Disorders, Fourth Edition, Text Revision.* Washington DC: American Psychiatric Publishing, Inc., 2000.

American Society for Bariatric Surgery. 100 S.W. 75th St. Suite 201. Gainesville, FL 32607. www.asbs.org.

Armitage A. Motivating overweight adults to lose weight. *Clinical Excellence for Nurse Practitioners* 2003;7(4):92–8.

Armstrong CA, Sallis JF, Hovell M, Hofsetter CR. Stages of change, self-efficacy, and the adoption of vigorous exercise: A prospective analysis. *Journal of Sport & Exercise Psychology* 1993;15:390–402.

Baile WF, Engel BT. A behavioral strategy or promoting treatment compliance following myocardial infarction. *Psychosomatic Medicine* 1978;40:413–19.

Baker RC, Kirschenbaum DS. Weight control during the holidays: Highly consistent self-monitoring as a potentially useful coping mechanism. *Health Psychology* 1998;17(4).

Ball K, Lee C. Psychological stress, coping, and symptoms of disordered eating in a community sample of young Australian women. *International Journal of Eating Disorders* 2002;31(1):71–81.

Bandura A, Walters RH. *Social Learning and Personality Development.* New York: Holt, Rinehart, and Winston, 1963.

Bandura A, Simon KM. The role of proximal intentions in self-regulation of refractory behavior. *Cognitive Therapy and Research* 1977;1:177–93.

Bandura A. Self-efficacy: Toward a unifying theory of behavioral change. *Psychological Review* 1977;84:191–215.

Beck JS. *Cognitive Therapy: Basics and Beyond.* New York: Guilford Press, 1995.

Benotti PN, Forse RA. The role of gastric surgery in the multidisciplinary management of severe obesity. *The American Journal of Surgery* 1995;169:361–7.

Bittinger JN, Smith JE. Mediating and moderating effects of stress perception and situational coping responses in women with disordered eating. *Eating Behaviors* 2003;4(1):89–1–6.

Blaine BE, DiBlasi DM, Connor JM. The effect of weight loss on perceptions of weight controllability: Implications for prejudice against overweight people. *Journal of Applied Biobehavioral Research* 2002;7(1):44–56.

Blaine B, Williams Z. Belief in the controllability of weight and attributions to prejudice against heavyweight women. *Sex Roles* 2004;51(1–2):79–84.

Boon B, Stroebe W, Schut H. Food for thought: Cognitive regulation of food intake. *British Journal of Health Psychology* 1998;3:27–40.

Booth DA, Blair AJ, Lewis VJ, Baek SH. Patterns of eating and movement that best maintain reduction in overweight. *Appetite* 2004;43(3):277–83.

Brownell KD. Behavioral medicine. In: Franks CM, Wilson GT, Kendall P, Brownell KD (eds). *Annual Review of Behavior Therapy: Theory and Practice. Volume Eight.* New York: Guildford Press, 1982.

Brownell KD, Foreyt JP (eds). *The Handbook of Eating Disorders. Physiology, Psychology and Treatment of Obesity, Anorexia, and Bulimia.* New York: Basic Books, HarperCollins Publishers, 1986.

Brownell KD. *The LEARN Program for Weight Control.* Dallas, TX: Brownell & Hager, 1989.

Buffington CK. Alcohol and the gastric bypass patient. *Bariatric Times.* 2006;3(8):1,8–10.

Buffington CK. Alcohol use and health risks survey results. *Bariatric Times.* 2007;4(2):1,21–23.

Byrne SM. Psychological aspects of weight maintenance and relapse in obesity. *Journal of Psychosomatic Research* 2002;53(5):1029–36.

Byrne S, Cooper Z, Fairburn C. Weight maintenance and relapse in obesity: A qualitative study. *International Journal of Obesity and Related Metabolic Disorders* 2003;27(8):955–62.

Byrne SM, Cooper Z, Fairburn CG. Psychological predictors of weight regain in obesity. *Behaviour Research and Therapy* 2004;42(11):1341–56.

Camerini G, Adami GF, Marinari G, et al. Satiety after vertical banded gastroplasty. *Eating and Weight Disorders* 2003;8(1):80–3.

Camps M, Zervos E, Goode S, Rosemurgy A. Impact of bariatric surgery on body image perception and sexuality in morbidly obese patients and their partners. *Obesity Surgery.* 2006;6(4):356–360.

Carels RA, Douglass OM, Cacciapaglia HM, O'Brien WH. An ecological momentary assessment of relapse crises in dieting. *Journal of Consulting & Clinical Psychology* 2004;72(2):341–8.

Castellani W, Ianni L, Ricca V, et al. Adherence to structured physical exercise in overweight and obese: A review of psychological models. *Eating and Weight Disorders* 2003;8(1):1–11.

Castelnuovo-Tedesco P, Douglas S. Studies of superobesity II. Psychiatric appraisal of jejuno-ileal bypass surgery. *American Journal of Psychiatry* 1976;133(1):26–31.

Claiborn J, Pedrick CT. *The Habit Change Workbook: How to Break Bad Habits and Form Good Ones.* Oakland, CA: New Harbinger Publications, Inc., 2001.

Cossrow NHF, Jeffery RW, McGuire MT. Understanding weight stigmatization: A focus group study. *Journal of Nutrition Education* 2001;33(4):208–14.

Davis M, Eshelman E, McKay M. *The Relaxation and Stress Reduction Workbook, Fifth Edition.* Oakland, CA: New Harbinger Publications, Inc., 2000.

Delin CR, Anderson PG. A preliminary comparison of the psychological impact of laparoscopic gastric banding and gastric bypass surgery for morbid obesity. *Obesity Surgery* 1999;9:155–60.

Dittman M. Weighing in on fat bias. *Monitor on Psychology.* American Psychological Association, 2004;35(1).

Dohm FA, Beattie JA, Aibel C, Striegel-Moore RH. Factors differentiating women and men who successfully maintain weight loss from women and men who do not. *Journal of Clinical Psychology* 2001;57(1):105–17.

Drapkin RG, Wing RR, Shiffman S. Responses to hypothetical high risk situations: Do they predict weight loss in a behavioral treatment program or the context of dietary lapses? *Health Psychology* 1995;14(5):427.

Dymek MP, Le Grange D, Neven K, Alverdy J. Quality of life and psychosocial adjustment in patients after roux-en-y gastric bypass: A brief report. *Obesity Surgery* 2004;11(1):32–9.

Epstein L, Cluss P. A behavioral medicine perspective on adherence to long-term medical regimens. *Journal of Consulting and Clinical Psychology* 1982;50:950–71.

Eton DT. Social support and its relation to weight control: An empirical analysis. *Dissertation Abstracts International: Section B—The Sciences & Engineering* 1999;59(11-B):6115.

Fobi MAL. Surgical treatment of obesity: A review. *Journal of the National Medical Association* 2004;96(1):61–75.

Foreyt JP, Goodrick GK. Attributes of successful approaches to weight loss and control. *Applied and Preventive Psychology* 1994;3(4):209–15.

Foreyt JP, Goodrick GK. Factors common to successful therapy for the obese patient. *Medicine and Science in Sports and Exercise* 1991;23(3):292–7.

Foster GD, Wadden TA, Vogt RA. Body image in obese women before, during, and after weight loss treatment. *Health Psychology* 1997;16(3).

Freeman LM, Gil KM. Daily stress, coping, and dietary restraint in binge eating. *International Journal of Eating Disorders* 2004;36(2):204–12.

Gauron EF. *Mental Training for Peak Performance.* Lansing, NY: Sport Science Associates, 1984.

Gauvin L. An experiential perspective on the motivational features of exercise and lifestyle. *Canadian Journal of Sport Sciences* 1990;15:51–8.

Glinski J, Wetzler S, Goodman E. The psychology of gastric bypass surgery. *Obesity Surgery* 2001;11:581–8.

Golay A, Buclin S, Ybarra J, et al. New interdisciplinary cognitive-behavioural-nutritional approach to obesity treatment: A 5-year follow-up study. *Eating and Weight Disorders* 2004;9(1):29–34.

Gorin AA, Phelan S, Hill JO, Wing RR. Medical triggers are associated with better short- and long-term weight outcomes. *Preventive Medicine: An International Journal Devoted to Practice and Theory* 2004;39(3).

Gorin AA, Phenlan S, Wing RR, Hill JO. Promoting long-term weight control: Does dieting consistency matter? *International Journal of Obesity and Related Metabolic Disorders* 2004;28(2):278–81.

Green CG, Wing RR. Stress-induced eating. *Psychological Bulletin* 1994;115(3).

Grilo CM, Shiffman S, Wing R. Relapse crises and coping among dieters. *Journal of Consulting and Clinical Psychology* 1989;57(4):488–95.

Grilo CM, Shiffman S. Longitudinal investigation of the abstinence violation effect in binge eating. *Journal of Consulting and Clinical Psychology* 1994;62(3):611–19.

Grilo M. The assessment and treatment of binge eating disorders. *Journal of Practical Psychiatry and Behavioral Health* 1998;4:191–201.

Guisado JA, Vaz FJ, Lopez-Ibor MI, et al. Gastric surgery and restraint from food as triggering factors of eating disorders in morbid obesity. *International Journal of Eating Disorders* 2002;31(1):97–100.

Guisado JA, Vaz FJ, Alarcon J, et al. Psychopathological status and interpersonal functioning following weight loss in morbidly obese patients undergoing bariatric surgery. *Obesity Surgery* 2004;12(6):835–40.

Guisado JA, Vaz FJ. Psychopathological differences between morbidly obese binge eaters and non-binge eaters after bariatric surgery. *Eating and Weight Disorders* 2003;8(4):315–18.

Hafner RJ, Rogers J, and Watts JM. Psychological status before and after gastric restriction as predictors of weight loss in the morbidly obese. *Journal of Psychosomatic Research* 1990;34(3):295–302.

Harris DV, Harris BL. *The Athlete's Guide to Sport Psychology: Mental Training for Physical People.* New York: Leisure Press, 1984.

Head S, Brookhart A. Lifestyle modification and relapse prevention training during treatment for weight loss. *Behavior Therapy* 1997;28(2):307–21.

Hergenhahn BR, Olson MH. *An Introduction to Theories of Learning, Sixth Edition.* Upper Saddle River, NJ: Prentice Hall, 2001.

Hitchcock P, Pugh JA. Management of overweight and obese adults. *British Medical Journal* 2002;325:757–61.

Hsu LKG, Benotti PN, Dwyer J, et al. Nonsurgical factors that influence the outcome of bariatric surgery: A review. *Psychosomatic Medicine* 1998;60(3):338–46.

Jacobson E. The origins and development of progressive relaxation. *Journal of Behavior Therapy & Experimental Psychiatry* 1977;8(2):119–23.

Jacobson E. *Progressive Relaxation.* Chicago, IL: University of Chicago Press, 1938.

Jakicic JM, Clark K, Coleman E, et al. Appropriate intervention strategies for weight loss and prevention of weight regain for adults. *Medicine and Science in Sports and Exercise* 2001;33(12):2145–56.

Janis IL, Mann L. *Decision Making: A Psychological Analysis of Conflict, Choice and Commitment.* New York: Free Press, 1977.

Kalarchian MA, Terence WG, Brolin RE, Bradley L. Binge eating in bariatric surgery patients. *International Journal of Eating Disorders* 1998;23(1):89–92.

Kalarchian MA, Marcus MD. Management of the bariatric surgery patient: Is there a role for the cognitive behavior therapist? *Cognitive and Behavioral Practice* 2003;10:112–19.

Kalarchian M, Marcus M, Levine M. Psychiatric disorders among bariatric surgery candidates: relationship to obesity and functional health status. *American Journal of Psychiatry.* 2007;164(2):328–34.

King TK, Clark MM, Pera V. History of sexual abuse and obesity treatment outcome. *Addictive Behaviors* 1996;21(3):283–90.

Kirschenbaum DS, Dykman BM. Disinhibited eating by resourceful restrained eaters. *Journal of Abnormal Psychology* 1991;100(2):227–30.

Korotitsch WJ, Nelson-Gray RO. An overview of self-monitoring research in assessment and treatment. *Psychological Assessment* 1999;11(4):415.

Kraft AM. Weight loss and depression. *American Journal of Psychiatry* 1991;148(7):947–8.

Kumar N, Singh JG. A study of surgical stress among female patients. *Journal of Personality and Clinical Studies* 2001;17(2);100–7.

Laitinen J, Ek E, Sovio U. Stress-related eating and drinking behavior and body mass index as predictors of this behavior. *Preventative Medicine: An International Journal Devoted to Practice and Theory* 2002;34(1).

Larimer JE, Palmer RS, Marlatt GA. Relapse prevention: An overview of Marlatt's cognitive-behavioral model. *Alcohol Research and Health* 1999;23(2):151–60.

Lewis VJ, Blair AJ, Booth DA. Outcome of group therapy for body-image emotionality and weight-control self-efficacy. *Behavioural Psychotherapy* 1992;20:155–65.

Lemont D, Moorehead M, Parish M, Reto C, Ritz S Suggestions for the pre-surgical psychological assessment of bariatric surgery candidates. American Society for Metabolic and Bariatric Surgery. 2004. www.asmbs.org.

Levine MD, Kalarchian MA, Courcoulason A, Wisinski M, Marcus M. History of smoking and postcessation weight gain among weight loss surgery candidates. *Addictive Behavior*. 2007;32(10):2365–2371.

Locke EA, Lathan GP. *A Theory of Goal Setting and Task Performance.* Englewood Cliffs, NJ: Prentice Hall, 1990.

Logue AW. Evolutionary theory and the psychology of eating (1998). Access date: March 28, 2005. Available at: darwin.baruch.cuny.edu/faculty/LogueA.html.

Marcoux BC, Trenkner LL, Rosenstock IM. Social networks and social support in weight loss. *Patient Education and Counseling* 1990;15(3):229–38.

Marcus JD, Elkins GR. Development of a model for a structured support group for patients following bariatric surgery. *Obesity Surgery* 2004;14:103–6.

Marcus JD, Elkins GR. Laparoscopic adjustable gastric band: Do support groups add to the weight loss? *Obesity Surgery* 2004;14(8):1139–40.

Marlatt GA, Gordon J. *Relapse Prevention: Maintenance Strategies in Addictive Behavior Change.* New York: Guilford Press, 1985.

Martin JE, Dubbert PM, Katell AD, et al. Behavior control of exercise in sedentary adults: Studies 1–6. *Journal of Consulting and Clinical Psychology* 1984;52:795–811.

McElroy SL, Kotwal R, Shishuka M, et al. Are mood disorders and obesity related? A review for the mental health profession. *Journal of Clinical Psychiatry* 2004;65(5):634–51.

McGuire MT, Wing RR, Klem ML, et al. What predicts weight regain in a group of successful weight losers. *Journal of Consulting & Clinical Psychology* 1999;67(3).

Meichenbaum D. *Cognitive-Behavior Modification.* New York: Plenum, 1977.

Miller CT, Rothblum ED, Felicio D, Brand P. Compensating for stigma: Obese and nonobese women's reactions to being visible. *Personality and Social Psychology Bulletin* 1995;21(10):1093–106.

Mitchell JE, deZwan M (eds). *Bariatric Surgery: A Guide for Mental Health Professionals.* New York, NY: Routledge, 2005.

Mooney JP, Burling TA, Hartman WM, Brenner-Liss D. The abstinence violation effect and very low calorie diet success. *Addictive Behaviors* 1992;17(4):319–24.

Moorehead M, Alexander C. Transfer of addiction and considerations for preventive measures in bariatric surgery (part 1). *Bariatric Times*, 2007;4(1) 22–25. (part 2) 2007;4(3)1, 18–21.

Musher-Eizenman DR, Holub SC, Miller AB, et al. Body size stigmatization in preschool children: The role of control in attributions. *Journal of Pediatric Psychology* 2004;29(8):613–20.

Myers AW, Schleser RA. A cognitive-behavioral intervention for improving basketball performance. *Journal of Sport Psychology* 1980;3:69–73.

National Eating Disorder Association. 603 Stewart Street, Suite 803, Seattle, WA 98101 www.nationaleatingdisorders.org.

National Institute of Mental Health. 6001 Executive Blvd. Room 8184, Bethesda, MD 20892 www.nimh.nih.gov.

National Strength and Conditioning Association. 1955 N. Union Blvd., Colorado Springs, CO 80909. www.nsca-lift.org.

Nejad LM, Wertheim EH, Greenwood KM. Predicted dieting behavior by using, modifying, and extending the theory of planned behavior. *Journal of Applied Social Psychology* 2004;34(10):2099–131.

Nickels R, Sayeed S, Sax HC. Predicting success after gastric bypass: The role of psychosocial and behavioral factors. *Surgery* 2003;134(4):555–63.

O'Connor DB, O'Connor RC. Perceived changes in food intake in response to stress: The role of conscientiousness. *Stress and Health: Journal of the International Society for the Investigation of Stress* 2004;20(5):279–91.

Ogden J, Whyman C. The effect of repeated weighing on psychological state. *European Eating Disorders Review.* 1997;5(2):121–30.

Ogden J, Wardle J. Control of eating and attributional style. *British Journal of Clinical Psychology* 1990;29(4):445–6.

Omalu, B, Ives, D, Buhari A et al. Death rates and causes of death after bariatric surgery for Pennsylvania residents. 1995-2004. *Archives of Surgery.* 2007;142(10) 923–928.

Passamonti L, Rowe JB, Schwarzbauer C, Ewbank MP, von dem Hagen E, Calder AJ. Personality predicts the brain's response to viewing appetizing foods. The neural basis of a risk factor for overeating. 2009;29(1):43–51.

Pavlov IP. *Conditioned Reflexes.* London: Oxford University Press, 1927.

Perri MG, Martin AD, Leermakers EA, et al. Effects of group versus home based exercise in the treatment of obesity. *Journal of Consulting and Clinical Psychology* 1997;65(2).

Perri MG, Nezu AM, McKelvey WF, Shermer RL. Relapse prevention training and problem-solving therapy in the long-term management of obesity. *Journal of Consulting and Clinical Psychology* 2001;69(4):722.

Polivy J, Herman CP, McFarlane T. Effects of anxiety on eating: Does palatability moderate distress-induced overeating in dieters? *Journal of Abnormal Psychology* 1994;103(30):505–10.

Porter LC, Wampler RS. Adjustment to rapid weight loss. *Families, Systems, and Health* 2000;18(1):35–54.

President's Council on Physical Fitness and Sports. Dept. W, 200 Independence Ave, SW, Room 738-H. Washington, DC 20201 www.fitness.gov.

Prochaska JO, DiClemente CC. Transtheoretical therapy: Toward a more integrative model of change. *Psychotherapy: Theory, Research and Practice* 1982;19:276–88.

Raglin JS. Exercise and mental health: Beneficial and detrimental effects. *Sports Medicine* 1990;9:323–9.

Rich LE. Along with increased surgery, a growing need for support. American Psychological Association: *Monitor on Psychology* 2004;35(1).

Rosenstock IM. Historical origins of the health belief model. *Health Education Monographs* 1966;2:323–9.

Saunders R, Johnson L, Teschner J. Prevalence of eating disorders among bariatric surgery patients. *Eating Disorders: The Journal of Treatment & Prevention* 1998;6(4):309–17.

Saunders R. Compulsive eating and gastric bypass surgery: What does hunger have to do with it? *Obesity Surgery* 2001;11:757–61.

Saunders R. "Grazing:" A high-risk behavior. *Obesity Surgery* 2004;14:98–102.

Schwartz MB, Brownell KD. Obesity and body image. *Body Image* 2003;1:43–56.

Sjostrom L, Lindroos A, Peltonen M, et al. Lifestyle, diabetes, and cardiovascular risk factors 10 years after bariatric surgery. *New England Journal of Medicine* 2004;351(26):2683–93.

Skinner BF. *Science and Human Behavior.* New York: Macmillan, 1953.

Solomon CG, Dluhy RG. Bariatric surgery: Quick fix or long term solution? *New England Journal of Medicine* 2004;351(26):2751–3.

Song A, Rubin J, Thomas V et al. Body image and quality of life in post massive weight loss body contouring patients. *Obesity.* 2006;14(9); 1626–36.

Stunkard AJ, Faith MS, Allison KC. Depression and obesity. *Biological Psychiatry* 2003;54(3):330–7.

Wadden TA, Stunkard AJ (eds). *Handbook of Obesity Treatment.* New York, NY, Guilford Press, 2002.

Wadden TA, Sarwer DB, Womble LG, et al. Psychosocial aspects of obesity and obesity surgery. *Obesity Surgery* 2001;81(5):1001–24.

Wallis DJ, Hetherington MM. Stress and eating: The effects of ego-threat and cognitive demand on food intake in restrained and emotional eaters. *Appetite* 2004;43:39–46.

Ward A, Mann T. Don't mind if I do: Disinhibited eating under cognitive load. *Journal of Personality and Social Psychology* 2000;78(4).

Weinberg RS, Weigand D. Goal setting in sport and exercise. A reaction to Locke. *Journal of Sport & Exercise Psychology* 1993;15:88–95.

Williams P, Lord S. Predictors of adherence to a structured exercise program for older women. *Psychology and Aging* 1995;10(4).

Wooley SC, Wooley OW, Dyrenforth SR. Theoretical, practical, and social issues in behavioral treatments of obesity. *Journal of Applied Behavior Analysis* 1979;12:3–25.

Yalom ID. *Theory and Practice of Group Psychotherapy.* New York: BasicBooks. A Division of HarperCollins Publishers, Inc., 1995.

Zarabi S. Exercise…the key to weight loss success. *Bariatric Times.* 2008;5(10):27–32.